WM224

State of the art in dementia care

edited by Mary Marshall

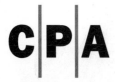

First published in 1997
by the Centre for Policy on Ageing
25-31 Ironmonger Row
London EC1V 3QP

© 1997 Centre for Policy on Ageing

British Library Cataloguing in Publication Data
A catalogue record for this book is available from
the British Library.

ISBN 0-904139-99-9

Designed by Jeremy Austen
Printed by Geerings, Ashford, Kent

The cover photograph is reproduced with kind
permission of Mrs Rose Kirk and Miss Margaret
Kennedy. Miss Kennedy is a carer with the adult
placement scheme run by the Falkirk, Stirling and
Clackmannan Joint Dementia Initiative. Mrs Kirk
lives with her. They are delighted to be on the
cover of this book and hope that adult placements
for people with dementia will be set up
elsewhere. It has been a very good experience for
them both. A report on the adult placement
scheme is published by the Dementia Services
Development Centre.

Contents

About the contributors   vii

Introduction: state of the art in dementia care. *Mary Marshall*   xiii

Part one
Listening to people with dementia and their carers   1

1 Collaboration and interdependence: care as a two-way street.
Elizabeth Barnett   1

2 In sickness and in health: remembering the relationship in family
caregiving for people with dementia. *Charlotte L Clarke*   7

3 Insight and dementia. *Andrew Fairbairn*   13

4 Between a rock and a hard place: the impact of dementia on
young carers. *Jane Gilliard*   18

5 Hearing the voice of people with dementia. *Malcolm Goldsmith*   22

6 Maintaining involvement: a meta concept to describe the
dynamics of dementia. *John Keady*   25

7 Confidences: the experience of writing with people
with dementia. *John Killick*   32

8 The uniqueness of persons in dementia. *Tom Kitwood*   36

9 Why should family caregivers feel guilty? *Robert T Woods*   39

Part two
Policies and services   45

10 Social Services Inspectorate inspection of services for older people
with dementia in the community. *Derek Brown*   45

11 EACH: European Alzheimer Clearing House. *Leen Meulenbergs*   46

12 Taking dementia services in Victoria into the twenty-first century.
Rosemary Calder   48

13 The art of the state: public policy in dementia care. *Harry Cayton*   54

14 Pragmatic groups: interactions and relationships between people
with dementia. *Kate Foster*   57

15 Staff issues in the hospital and in the community: a case for
    retaining longstay hospital provision. *Alan Gilloran*   62

16 Problems in recognising dementia in general practice: how can
    they be overcome? *Steve Iliffe*   67

17 Old age psychiatry and dementia: somebody cares. *David Jolley* 73

18 Group homes: an alternative for older people with dementia.
    Bo Malmberg   78

19 Personal finances and elderly people with dementia: a challenge
    for local authorities. *Robin Means*   83

20 Home based respite care. *Sue Newton*   89

21 Elder abuse and dementia: moving forward. *Lynne Phair*   91

22 Advocacy and older people with dementia. *Andrew Dunning*   95

Part three
Working together   102

23 Bounce and balance: a team approach to risk management for
    people with dementia living at home. *April Baragwanath*   102

24 Joint working: the impossible dream? *Valerie Good*   106

25 Which hat should we wear today? Recruiting and developing
    the ideal workforce for dementia care. *Gill Herbert*   111

26 Demolishing the barriers: community dementia team development
    in Coventry. *David Sheard*   116

27 Dementia care management: healing the split. *Phyllis J Sturges* 123

Part four
Interventions   129

28 Therapies in old age psychiatry: reflections on recent changes.
    Susan M Benbow   129

29 Owning the past in dementia care: creative engagement with others
    in the present. *Faith Gibson*   134

30 Neuroleptic prescribing in dementia: uses, problems and
    ethical issues. *Graham Jackson*   139

31 Technology. *Stephen Judd*   144

32 Life story work. *Charlie Murphy and Marion Moyes*   149

33 What do we mean when we talk about assessment? *Gregor McWalter* 154

34 Rewriting the story of dementia: a narrative approach to psychotherapy with people with dementia.
Laura J Sutton and Richard Cheston 159

Part five
Buildings, fixtures and fittings 164

35 Cultural issues in designing for people with dementia. *Kirsty Bennett* 164

36 'A journey with Alice'. *Brian J Kidd* 169

37 Mealtime experiences. *Lesley Malone* 175

38 'You're sitting in my chair': an enquiry into the role and function of appropriate seating for the active person with dementia.
Gretta Peachment 178

Part six
Training 183

39 Is multidisciplinary training possible? *Alan Chapman* 183

40 Sir James McCusker Training Foundation: developing a dementia care consultancy service. *Beth Douglas* 188

Part seven
Younger people with dementia 193

41 Younger people with dementia: challenging the system. *Sylvia Cox* 193

42 HIV related dementia: the benefits of a small homely environment with a holistic client-centred approach. *Buz de Villiers* 198

Part eight
The media 204

43 Alzheimer in Ballarat. *Tom Arie* 204

44 Cinderella's rag: refreshing the parts other journals cannot reach.
Sue Benson 205

Part nine
Evaluation and critique 207

45 Evaluating dementia services. *Murna Downs* 207

46 The continuing quest for predictors of breakdown of family care of elderly people with dementia. *Pauline Lightbody and Mary Gilhooly* 211

Part ten
Sex, death and spirituality 217

47 Sexuality and dementia? *Carole Archibald* 217

48 Talking about death. *Mary Dixon* 221

49 Spiritual needs and religious practice in dementia care. *Alison Froggatt and Laraine Moffitt* 225

50 From factory to hearth: valuing humanness in dementia care. *Monica Nebauer and Kim Wylie* 230

Index 236

About the contributors

Carole Archibald BA (Hons) RGN, HV is Senior Fieldworker at the Dementia Services Development Centre, University of Stirling and has worked in the field of dementia care for twelve years. Her interests include activities for people with dementia, respite care, specialist dementia units and sexuality.

Tom Arie CBE, FRCP, FRCPsych is the Foundation Professor Emeritus of Health Care of the Elderly, University of Nottingham. He is a Governor of the Centre for Policy on Ageing.

Elizabeth Barnett's background is in health service management and research. She has recently completed her PhD in social policy. At present she works as a freelance Trainer and Consultant in dementia care and is an Associate of the Bradford Dementia Group.

Dr Susan Benbow MD, ChB, MSC, FRCPsych, Dip Fam Ther is a Consultant in Old Age Psychiatry at Central Manchester NHS Trust and for the past nine months has been on secondment to the West Cheshire Trust setting up an old age psychiatry service for Chester, Ellesmore Port and part of Cheshire.

April Baragwanath is a social worker and currently General Manager, Community Care with St Laurence Community Services (Barwon) Inc in Victoria, Austalia. She was awarded the 1994 Sir Vincent Fairfax Churchill Fellowship to study community care programmes for people with dementia in the USA, Canada and UK.

Kirsty Bennett BArch(Hons), GradDipGer is Associate Director at Kerr Lewit Clark and Kidd, Architects in Melbourne, Western Australia.

Sue Benson BA(Hons), RGN is editor of the *Journal of Dementia Care*.

Derek Brown is an Inspector with the Social Services Inspectorate, Gateshead. Most of his career has been concerned with services for people with dementia.

Rosemary Calder has been Manager of Aged Services Redevelopment in the Department of Human Services in Melbourne, Australia since 1995 and has been responsible for policy and strategic development of State-funded residential, specialist acute, rehabilitation and other health services for older people since 1990.

Harry Cayton BA, BPhil, DipAnth is Executive Director of the Alzheimer's Disease Society. He has family experience of caring for someone with dementia. He has written and spoken widely on ethical and policy issues in health and social care.

Alan Chapman is responsible for the training service at the Dementia Services Development Centre, University of Stirling. He orginally trained and worked as a social worker and since joining the Centre in 1991 he has written and edited a number of training publications, as well as leading training with multidisciplinary groups of staff.

Dr Richard Cheston is a Lecturer in Psychology at the School of Social Sciences, University of Bath. He also works as a Clinical Psychologist working with older people for the Weston Area Health Trust in Weston-super-Mare.

Dr Charlotte Clarke RGN, BA, MSc, PGCE, PhD is a Research Fellow at the Faculty of Health, Social Work and Education, University of Northumbria at Newcastle. She has previously worked in clinical posts with older people and in the education of health care professionals. Research activity includes dementia care, family caring and the processes of developing health care practice.

Sylvia Cox is Planning Consultant with the Dementia Services Development Centre, University of Stirling. She is a qualified social worker and has worked as a practitioner and senior manager. She held the post of Principal Officer for Community Care in Strathclyde Regional Social Work Department for a number of years and is also a member of the Scottish Health Advisory Service.

Murna Downs PhD is currently Research Manager at the Dementia Services Development Centre, University of Stirling. Recent work examines the relocation of staff caring for people with dementia from hospital to the community and the role of primary care in dementia diagnosis and management.

Mary Dixon is currently employed as a Specialist Social Worker working with older people for Falkirk Council. She has held a variety of social work posts since beginning her career in 1977 and has a particular interest in working with people with dementia.

Beth Douglas is Director of the Sir James McCusker Training Project in Western Australia. The Foundation's multidisciplinary team has been developing, delivering and evaluating a range of dementia specific training packages throughout Western Australia for six years and, in the past six months, in Queensland.

Andrew Dunning is a Policy Officer at the Centre for Policy on Ageing and author of *Citizen Advocacy with Older People: a code of good practice* (CPA). He has previously worked as a social worker, lecturer and coordinator of a citizen advocacy project.

Dr Andrew Fairbairn is an Old Age Psychiatrist based at the Institute for Health of the Elderly at Newcastle-upon-Tyne, currently seconded half-time to the Department of Health.

Alison Froggatt retired from being a Lecturer in Social Work at Bradford University and has been associated with the Bradford Dementia Research Group. She is Secretary of the Christian Council on Ageing Dementia Working Group

Kate Foster is a PhD student at the Dementia Services Development Centre, University of Stirling. Her thesis is an evaluation of specialist care housing. Previous research work has included evaluation of day care for younger people with dementia.

Faith Gibson is Professor of Social Work at the University of Ulster in Northern Ireland. Her ideas about dementia have been influenced by experience as reminiscence practitioner, teacher, researcher and family carer.

Mary Gilhooly PhD is Professor of Health Studies and Director of the Centre of Gerontology and Health Studies at the University of Paisley. Current areas of research include family care of elderly people with dementia, unreported accidents amongst the elderly living at home and the role of community nurses in the social networks of carers of mentally disordered old people.

Jane Gilliard is a Research Fellow at the School for Policy Studies, University of Bristol where her research interests include counselling support for people with dementia and their carers, the experience of people in the early stages of dementia and the impact of dementia on young carers. Jane has written the only book to date aimed specifically at informing young people about dementia.

Alan Gilloran MA, PhD is currently Senior Lecturer in Sociology and Social Policy at Queen Margaret College, Edinburgh. His main areas of reseach include work satisfaction and the quality of care in hospital wards for people with dementia, the relocation of staff caring for people with dementia to the community, and culture change in mental health care.

Malcolm Goldsmith is a clergyman in Edinburgh. He has worked as a research fellow at the Dementia Services Development Centre at the University of Stirling and maintains close contact there. He is the author of *Hearing the Voice of People with Dementia*.

Valerie Good has spent the last sixteen years working with older people with dementia in a variety of settings. She is particularly interested in the development of services and the application of new technology and research.

She is currently employed as a Service Development Manager for Anchor Trust.

Gill Herbert has spent many years designing, developing and managing community services for people with dementia within health and social services and the independent sector. She is now a Development Consultant at the Nuffield Institute for Health at Leeds University in the Community Care Division.

Steve Iliffe MRCGP is a General Practitioner in northwest London and Reader in Primary Health Care, Department of Primary Health Care and Population Sciences at University College London Medical School.

David Jolley MSc, FRCPsych, Professor in Old Age Psychiatry, was appointed as the first Old Age Psychiatrist in the North West Region in 1975 developing services, training and research. He is currently Medical Director of the Community Trust in Wolverhampton responsible for developing mental health and other services in conjunction with the University of Wolverhampton.

Dr Stephen Judd is Chief Executive of the Hammond Care Group which is based in Sydney, Australia. Hammond Care exists to nurture dignity and improve the quality of life for older people and dementia sufferers, especially those least able to provide for themselves. Stephen has worked in both the health care and information technology industries.

Graham A Jackson MRCPsych, MRCGP is a Senior Registrar in Old Age Psychiatry in the west of Scotland. He is a former GP. His interests include expanding psychiatric care into non-hospital environments.

John Keady is a Lecturer in Nursing at the University of Wales, Bangor. Working closely with Professor Mike Nolan at the University of Sheffield, he has undertaken a study which explores both the experience of caring at home for a person with dementia and the experience of dementia itself.

Brian J Kidd AM, MArch, FRAIA is a Senior Associate, Faculty of Architecture and Planning, the University of Melbourne, and Director, Kerr Lewit Clark and Kidd Architects.

John Killick works as a writer for Westminster Health Care, and also for the Dementia Services Development Centre, University of Stirling, who published his account of his methods *Please Give Me Back My Personality!* in 1994. *YOU ARE WORDS: Dementia Poems* is forthcoming from Hawker Publications.

Tom Kitwood is Leader of the Bradford Dementia Group. He has over ten years experience in working with and for people who have dementia and their carers. His particular concern is with the development of person-centred care.

Pauline Lightbody PhD is a research fellow at the Centre of Gerontology and Health Studies at the University of Paisley.

Bo Malmberg PhD is Senior Researcher at the Institute of Gerontology, College of Health Sciences, Jönköping, Sweden and Assistant Professor at the Department of Biobehavioural Health and Human Development at the Pennsylvania State University, USA. His main interests are social psychological gerontology and special forms of accommodation for older people.

Lesley Malone BSc, MPhil is a Clinical Psychologist. During her training she carried out a review of the literature on mealtimes and dementia for the Dementia Services Development Centre, University of Stirling.

Gregor McWalter is a Senior Health Information Scientist with the Information and Statistics Division Scotland, part of the National Health Service in Scotland. He was formerly Research Psychologist on a project which investigated needs assessment for people with dementia and their carers.

Robin Means is a Reader in Social Gerontology at the School for Policy Studies, University of Bristol. He has carried out extensive research in community care issues and is presently producing a workbook with colleagues for the Department of Health/Department of Environment on joint working at the operational level across housing, health and social services.

Leen Meulenbergs is the Project Manager at the European Alzheimer Clearing House in Brussels.

Laraine Moffitt is the worker for a project set up by the Christian Council on Ageing which is concerned with the spiritual needs of people with dementia and their carers. She has an Honours Degree in Religious Studies and is a Registered General Nurse.

Marion Moyes is a Charge Nurse of a day care facility, Gala Day Unit, for the Borders Community Health Services NHS Trust. She has had an interest in the development and promotion of life story work with people with dementia over a number of years.

Charlie Murphy has been Fieldworker for the voluntary sector with the Dementia Services Development Centre, University of Stirling since 1992. He is author of *It Started with a Sea-shell: Life Story Work with People with Dementia*, published by the Centre in 1991.

Monica Nebauer RN, EM, BAppSc(Nsg), MPhil Doctoral Candidate, University of Melbourne, Senior Lecturer at Australian Catholic University.

Sue Newton is Deputy Director of Liverpool Personal Service Society. She has been organising Adult Placement Services since 1978 and is Chairman of the National Association of Adult Placement Services.

Gretta Peachment BA, RN, Churchill Fellow 1996, Consultant for Facilities and Planning, Homes of Peace in Western Australia. As a Health Care Designer focusing on Dementia, Huntington's and Parkinson's disease she aims to ensure that buildings actively contribute to wellbeing.

Lynne Phair RMN, RGN,BSc(Hons), DPNS, PGCCC is the Team Leader Mental Health Services for Older People, Eastbourne and County Health Care NHS. She has a particular research interest in abuse of older people and has been part of a multidisciplinary group to develop guidelines for the protection of vulnerable adults in East Sussex.

David Sheard BA, CQSW is a freelance consultant in dementia care and mental health services. He was formerly General Manager of Old Age Psychiatry in Coventry with fifteen years experience across health and social services.

Dr Phyllis Sturges is a Lecturer at the School of Applied Social Studies, Robert Gordon University, Aberdeen. An American, she has been doing research for the past five years on the development of care management practice in Britain.

Dr Laura J Sutton is a Chartered Clinical Psychologist at the Western Community Hospital in Southampton. She has a special interest in working with survivors of past trauma in late life, in the development of psychotherapy with older people, including people with dementia.

Buz de Villiers is manager of FLAGS – a division of the St Mungo Community Trust. FLAGS operates Patrick House, a specialist nursing home for people with HIV related brain impairment. Buz was responsible for the development of Patrick House and for bringing it into management in 1992.

Bob Woods is Professor of Clinical Psychology of the Elderly,University of Wales, Bangor. His books include *Alzheimer's Disease: coping with a living death* and *Positive Approaches to Dementia Care* with Una Holden.

Kim Wylie RGN, RPN, BHSc(Nurs), MN Doctoral Candidate at the University of Newcastle, Churchill Fellow in 1993, is based in Australia.

Introduction: state of the art in dementia care

Mary Marshall

Dementia care is a very dynamic field to be in at present. This has not always been the case. Until ten or so years ago it was characterised by profound therapeutic nihilism. The combination of characteristics: old age, challenging behaviour, incompetence, loss of insight, low status, increasing numbers and poor success in pharmacological research cast a deep shadow. Much of dementia care still operates in this shadow but a much more optimistic and dynamic approach is becoming the norm. There are many possible reasons for this.

The first is the omnipresence of the disease in its various manifestations (Alzheimer's, Vascular, etc). Few people in the more developed countries have been untouched by it, either because they have it, fear they have it or are close to someone who has or has had it. The less developed countries face very substantial numbers of people with this disease in the next 20-30 years. Tom Arie's reflections in this book are about the extent to which the words Alzheimer's disease are now widely understood. This omnipresence means that many people are highly motivated, often by personal experience, to improve dementia care.

The second is the effective voice of carers. They have set up energetic and articulate organisations (Alzheimer's Disease Society and Alzheimer's Scotland Action on Dementia in the UK). Some of them have written moving accounts of their experiences either as non-fiction (Mace et al, 1992) or as fiction (Forster, 1989; Ignatieff, 1993).

People with dementia have, so far, been less vocal although at least two have written personal accounts (Davies, 1993; Friel McGowin, 1993). The degree of interest in John Killick's poetry (1994) seems to demonstrate increasing public interest. The poems in his chapter in this book will allow readers to judge whether they share his conviction that people with dementia are trying to communicate genuine feelings and opinions.

There has also been a burgeoning professional literature. Books on therapies such as reality orientation (Holden and Woods, 1988) and validation therapy (Feil, 1992) have been widely read. There have been books for social workers (Marshall, 1996; Chapman and Marshall, 1993), clinical psychology (Woods, 1996), occupational therapists (Conroy, 1996) and residential staff (Chapman et al, 1994). There have been a great many general texts for professionals, some written by psychiatrists (Jacques, 1992; Murphy, 1986) and some by nurses and social workers (for example Phair and Good, 1995) and psychologists (Stokes and Goudie, 1990). There are invaluable North American texts on running dementia units (Peppard, 1991; Hiatt, 1985; Coons, 1991).

Tom Kitwood's concept of a new culture of dementia care (Kitwood and Bredin, 1992; Kitwood and Benson, 1995) has been very influential across the board. The setting up of the Dementia Services Development Centre at the University of Stirling in 1989 represented a significant awareness of the importance of care as well as cure. The emergence of similar Centres in the Republic of Ireland, Newcastle, Bristol and Belfast will strengthen this focus. Equally significant has been the publication of the *Journal of Dementia Care*, which recognised the importance of shared expertise in this new field. Sue Benson's contribution demonstrates why this journal has been such a success.

This crescendo of interest is well illustrated by the increasing numbers of international, European, national and local conferences on dementia care. The world is a different place from the days when Tom Arie and the small number of like-minded enthusiasts stomped around the country (and the world) trying to stir up enthusiasm. David Jolley is one of this band and he demonstrates his own brand of pragmatic optimism in his chapter.

CPA itself has been very influential primarily through the work of Alison Norman (1987). It therefore seemed appropriate to publish a celebratory text about dementia care, illustrating its creativity and dynamism, in the year of CPA's golden jubilee. It was agreed that I would write to a large number of enthusiasts from many backgrounds and ask them to write a short piece about their current preoccupations. The time scale was very tight of necessity and design. The aim was to get fresh, personal and possibly speculative papers rather than accounts of well worn research. Many people asked were unable to provide a paper in the time. A surprising number were keen and provided exactly what was required. This is a rather larger book than we had anticipated.

Having got the papers the next issue was how to present them. They are a treasure box and we would have liked to maintain the element of surprise by simply mixing them up. However, on reflection, we decided to try and order them. This has its limitations because the papers do not fall into comfortable themes. The ordering is somewhat arbitrary and many could be in several of the sections. Perhaps this will sustain the sense of surprise and delight.

There are, of course, major gaps in this collection as a result of the way the pieces were collected. The contributors are all, but one, from the UK and Australia (the latter a recognition of CPA's link with Australia through the Warren sisters). North Americans are prolific publishers elsewhere so this is not a serious omission. The lack of contributions about dementia care in less developed countries is a serious omission which should be remedied in a second volume if this is possible. Related to this is the omission of any specific contribution on dementia care and minority ethnic groups. An Australian contributor mentions cultural sensitivity (see Kirsty Bennett's chapter) but it is an issue, with few exceptions, neglected by British contributors. This issue deserves urgent attention. There is a major gap in British literature as a whole.

The impression given by this collection, which I think is a true reflection of the state of the art, is the degree of attention given to listening to people with dementia and their carers. This is the largest section of the book and the papers have a special passion. Really listening is rare, listening to people with dementia as well as their carers is even more radical. This will fundamentally change our services over the next decade in my view. This is illustrated by Charlotte Clarke and Bob Woods who both emphasise the significance of relationships to which people adjust to accommodate the dementia. Professionals can tend to focus on the strain of the carer or on the dementia, often neglecting the importance of the relationship. Jane Gilliard draws attention to young people who are carers but whose feelings are often neglected, and John Keady describes the phases of adjustment people with dementia seem to go through.

There are remarkably few conflicting views in this set of papers. One of the few is the difference of opinion on the extent to which people in the later stages of dementia have something coherent to say. John Killick suggests a special language, whereas Andrew Fairbairn identifies a lack of insight; Elizabeth Barnett considers her research demonstrated awareness, if not insight, and Malcolm Goldsmith hints that we professionals may be unwilling to hear the voice of people with dementia because of the effect it may have on us. Their sources of evidence are different and, like the other papers in this section, should inform an ongoing debate.

The notion of a rationality retained, however impaired, is behind a great many papers. Indeed without this the interventions would be less meaningful. We can all accept that people with dementia have feelings but to hypothesise change and improvement has to suggest potential for intellectual change. No author spells this out. Perhaps they are instead suggesting that dementia care can avoid disabling people rather than actually rehabilitating them in the sense of restoring neurological function.

The section on policies and services is unsurprisingly a very mixed bag. Derek Brown, Rosemary Calder and Leen Meulenbergs share, in their papers, initiatives taken at national, state and European level to improve dementia services. Harry Cayton takes on a broad critique of social policy and dementia.

At the other end of the scale Kate Foster reflects on the practice of caring for people in small groups. I have often thought that group work skills should be taught to all of us so we are as successful as possible in making use of the services available to us in late life. Alan Gilloran's chapter underlines the likelihood that we may well end our days in longstay care if we get dementia, though he makes a strong case for better models of care.

Steve Iliffe and David Jolley have been very influential in their own professional fields of general practice and old age psychiatry. Here they demonstrate their approach. Steve Iliffe argues cogently for earlier diagnosis using research evidence. David Jolley movingly concludes his account of old age psychiatry with the assertion that people with dementia need services which 'own' them if despair is to be set aside.

Five relatively neglected areas of services are addressed by Bo Malmberg (care housing), Robin Means (personal finances), Sue Newton (home based respite), Lynne Phair (elder abuse) and Andrew Dunning (advocacy). They tackle their issues in different ways, but each underlines the importance of constantly reviewing services and constantly attempting to improve them. Numerous other neglected areas of service are not covered by this book, but these five papers illustrate how much we have yet to learn.

One area of service provision merited its own section: that of joint working. Five authors April Baragwanath, Valerie Good, Gill Herbert, David Sheard and Phyllis Sturges tackle it with vigour based on hard won experiences. The needs of people with dementia and their carers do not fall tidily into the health and welfare divide which characterises most systems of care in more developed countries. A great deal of professional time and energy is spent on meeting needs in spite of professional and structural boundaries. It is important to learn from others how to be as effective as possible.

A section on interventions might be expected to have a chapter on assessment and this one has (Gregor McWalter). Neuoleptic prescribing (Graham Jackson), reminiscence (Faith Gibson) and life story work (Charlie Murphy and Marion Moyes) might also be likely although perhaps not alongside each other. Susan Benbow's inclusion of psychotherapy along with Laura Sutton and Rik Cheston's paper on the subject might be thoroughly surprising. Psychotherapy with people with dementia is slowly taking its rightful place in the bank of possible interventions and it shows every sign of dynamic development, as does the field of technology (Stephen Judd). A more individualised and therapeutic approach to technology has considerable potential to improve the lives of people with dementia.

The built environment is highly significant for people with dementia. The more disabled a person is, the more significant the effect of the environment. People with dementia often lack the ability to make sense of, let alone modify the environment, so they need it to compensate for their disabilities. It is not insignificant that three of the authors in this section: Kirsty Bennett, Brian Kidd and Gretta Peachment are Australians. Brian Kidd, in particular, is a pioneer in designing for dementia and he has inspired both Kirsty Bennett and Gretta Peachment over the years. They have taken his thinking into new areas. Lesley

Malone, the remaining (Scottish) contributor provides an invaluable reflection on the importance of environment at mealtimes.

A book on the state of the art would have to have a section on training since training is a key to improving practice. Both Alan Chapman and Beth Douglas are very experienced trainers in the field of dementia care. Neither tackles the topic with a polemic about the importance of training; instead they share their experience in two different kinds of training.

Over the last five years the needs of young people with dementia have been recognised albeit as yet inadequately. Sylvia Cox provides an overview and Buz de Villiers shares his experience of working with one particular group in one project. Both emphasise the need for more resources.

Many of the contributors of this book are grounded in research but two papers address research itself. Pauline Lightbody and Mary Gilhooly review the research on predictors of family breakdown, and Murna Downs on issues of evaluation. There is a need for more writing which reviews research findings and identifies shortcomings and gaps, and presents what is known in an accessible form. Government determination to base practice on research should yield more work of this nature.

Sex, death and spirituality may seem like a dustbin concluding section, but the aim of clustering them is much more purposeful. These three topics are, in my view, barometers of the extent to which people with dementia are seen as people. If they are seen as people who have the capacity for sexual feelings and relationships, the capacity for bereavement and good death, and the capacity for spiritual feelings and growth then they are seen as being of equal humanity. Carole Archibald is well known for raising the issues of sexuality in a range of journals, books and conferences. Similarly Alison Froggatt and Laraine Moffitt have achieved a great deal on the issue of spirituality. Mary Dixon's paper is of a different order. She simply reflects on the experience of a family and how we might usefully be more aware of death and bereavement.

The book concludes with a passionate diatribe against much dementia care and for new holistic thinking. I would love to have been able to write a paper like this to conclude the book. Instead I am grateful to Monica Nebauer and Kim Wylie for doing it for me.

Tom Kitwood's influence is a strong one with many of the authors. His ability to communicate effectively about the basic humanity of people with dementia has been a very significant contribution to dementia and many authors were asked to remove substantial quotes from his work to avoid duplication. His chapter here about two preconditions for appreciating the uniqueness of individuals demonstrates his special skills.

I wish to record my thanks to this host of busy and dedicated people who so willingly contributed. And to Margaret Hope, the publications secretary at the Dementia Services Development Centre, who undertook all the really hard work in collecting, collating, reminding, checking and chasing. Many others have helped and to them also warm thanks. I hope this book enhances CPA's reputation of being in the vanguard of thinking about dementia and that it inspires many more activists in this field to put pen to paper and share their expertise.

References

Chapman A and Marshall M (eds) (1993) *Dementia: New Skills for Social Workers*. London: Jessica Kingsley Publishers.

Chapman A, Jacques A and Marshall M (1994) *Dementia Care: A Handbook forResidential and Day Care*. London: Age Concern.

Conroy MC (1996) *Dementia Care: Keeping Intact and In Touch*. Aldershot: Avebury.

Coons DH (1991) *Specialised Dementia Units*. Baltimore and London: The Johns Hopkins University Press.

Davies R (1993) *My Journey into Alzheimer's Disease*. Amersham-on-the-Hill: Scripture Press.

Feil N (1992) *Validation: The Feil Method*. Ohio: Edward Feil Productions.

Forster M (1989) *Have the Men Had Enough*. London: Chatto.

Friel McGowin D (1993) *Living in the Labyrinth: A Personal Journey Through the Maze of Alzheimer's*. USA: Elder Books.

Hiatt LG (1985) Understanding the Physical Environment. *Pride Institute Journal of Long Term Care* 4(2),12-22.

Holden UP and Woods RT (1988) *Reality Orientation: psychological approaches to the confused elderly*. London: Churchill Livingstone.

Ignatieff M (1993) *Scar Tissue: A Novel*. London: Chatto and Windus.

Jacques A (1992) (2nd Edition) *Understanding Dementia*. Edinburgh: Churchill Livingstone.

Killick J (1994) *Please Give Me Back My Personality! Writing and Dementia*. Stirling: Dementia Services Development Centre.

Kitwood T and Benson S (eds) (1995) *The New Culture of Dementia Care*. London: Hawker Publications.

Kitwood T and Bredin K (1992) (2nd Edition) *Person to Person: A Guide to the Care of Those with Failing Mental Powers*. Essex: Gale Centre Publications.

Kitwood T and Bredin K (1992) Toward a theory of dementia care: personhood and well-being. *Ageing and Society* 12, 269-287.

Mace NL, Rabins PV, Castleton BA, McEwan E and Meredith B (1992) *The 36 Hour Day*. London: Age Concern England.

Marshall M (1996) *'I Can't Place This Place At All': Working with People with Dementia and Their Carers*. Birmingham: Venture Press.

Murphy E (1986) *Dementia and Mental Illness in the Old*. London: Papermac.

Norman A (1987) *Severe Dementia – The Provision of Longstay Care*. London: CPA.

Peppard NR (1991) *Special Needs Dementia Units: Design, Development and Operations*. New York: Springer Publishing Company.

Phair L and Good V (1995) *Dementia: A Positive Approach*. London: Scutari Press.

Stokes G and Goudie F (1990) *Working with Dementia*. Bicester: Winslow Press.

Woods RT (ed) (1996) *Handbook of Clinical Psychology of Ageing*. Chichester: John Wiley.

Listening to people with dementia and their carers

1 Collaboration and interdependence: care as a two-way street

Elizabeth Barnett

> *People are brighter than we think...give them half a chance, they*
> *can be resourceful, they can be helpful... You don't have to bend*
> *down on people, not that at all, no. It's give and take.*
>
> 'James', client attending a day-hospital for elderly people with dementia

Care and collaboration

It is a truth (almost!) universally acknowledged that good practice in caring for elderly people with dementia must involve collaboration between the different disciplines and agencies concerned, and also family carers. But the service users themselves are still sidelined from the collaborative process. Elderly clients with dementia are seen as recipients of care and not as collaborators in the challenging task which their dementia presents to all concerned, including themselves.

This chapter explores the implications of this, drawing upon some of the findings of my doctoral research project, which evaluated care in a new facility specifically designed for elderly people with dementia. The research design was radical in that it was based on privileging the client perspective. I observed the apparent experience of clients in the unit using Dementia Care Mapping (Kitwood and Bredin, 1994), and I interviewed at length nearly all those involved with the unit – staff, managers, family carers, and two-thirds of the elderly people with dementia who used the service (some no longer communicated verbally at all). From analysing transcripts of the 'depth' interviews (Sutton, 1993) with the clients themselves their main concerns became clear, and it was these which I used to evaluate the service.

Insight and awareness

The usual reason given for not including people with dementia as equal partners in the care process is the claim that they 'lack insight'. However, 'insight' is so defined that people with dementia are almost inevitably excluded from possessing it, and moreover required to confess to being diseased (Jacques, 1988 pp183-187). Staff and managers interviewed spoke in terms of clients being more, or less, 'aware', but it was clear from what they said that this meant capable of coherent speech. This definition allowed them to divide those with whom they could still easily communicate verbally ('clients') from those with whom they could not ('patients'). Observation showed the implications of this division: that the quality of care experienced by a given individual varied in direct accordance with their verbal communication skills (see Figure 1.1).

Figure 1.1 Comparative experience of care of client groups differentiated by ability/disability to communicate verbally, measured by average individual care score

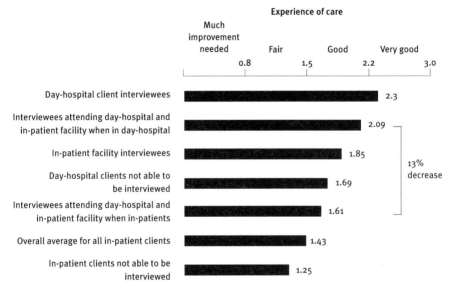

However, both my observational and interview data from service-users showed that, despite wide variation in verbal skills, all demonstrated awareness in different ways. For example, nearly half of those interviewed clearly demonstrated their awareness of the interview situation:

You're very welcome to ask me at any time for what I know might be very helpful. If there's anything you want to learn from me you're very welcome.

And a third of them spoke of their own confusion:

> *I haven't the foggiest notion, because I haven't got any notions.*
> *My problem is myself, have to remember. I forget, you see...*
> *I'm not much of a one to talk, because I don't know.*

How it can feel to be dependent on others

The interviews began with a single question: 'What is it like for you here at x?' As they considered this clients often related memory stories. I used narrative analysis of these to concentrate on their function in terms of the context. That is, 'Why this particular memory at this time (or position in the interview) and in this place x? What is the metaphorical meaning of this story?'

Many of these stories concerned childhood memories about their parents. Long term memories are more available to elderly people with dementia. But there are many other childhood memories than those involving parents. Given the context of the interview (always in the new unit) it seemed reasonable that the situation of dependence in which the clients again found themselves could be resuscitating other memories of dependence from their past. By analogy, then, the staff could be seen as being perceived in a parental role.

It was therefore disturbing that many of these memories were of strictness, and some even of abuse. These were memories of fear and impotent anger:

> *It used to be terrible... I've seen my Mum with many a black eye as*
> *a kid, and that all kept in your memory, you know, all that sort of*
> *thing. It did mine anyway. Me and my sisters we used to sit and cry*
> *to one another about it. 'What can we do?' we used to say...*
> *We can't do anything... I used to run away.*

Dependence for this client was therefore inherently frightening, probably the more so since she could no longer 'run away'.

Another client recounted memories of how his brothers had suffered in the 1914-18 war, and how his father (too old to fight but not looking his age) had been branded a coward by women in the street who pinned a white feather on him. This client was cared for at home by his daughter and in the unit almost exclusively by female staff. His other memories showed how strongly he had learned to value a patriarchal male role. For him, therefore, the experience of being dependent was, in itself, stigmatising.

Yet both these clients' *observed* experience of care was relatively good. Conversely, while both the staff and managers interviewed expressed great commitment to avoiding 'institutionalisation' (which, indeed, was their 'bogey word'!), for one client, the very fact of being again in an 'institution' revived very happy memories of school! In other words, however positive the present situation, for any given individual it seems the experience of being in a dependent role inevitably carries an emotional meaning informed by the past. With the best will in the world 'looking after' someone we unwittingly inherit an emotional legacy – and we cannot *assume* that it will be a positive one. All the more reason, therefore, for including the voice of the client in the care process.

Interdependence

The 'one-way street' of care, which proceeds from not recognising the awareness of clients with dementia, penalises them as their communication skills decrease, and excludes the crucial individual information which could support truly person-centred care. And by not listening to what clients themselves have to say we shut ourselves off from their wisdom. After all, they have known what it is like *not* to have dementia; the rest of us have not known what it is to have it.

The interview situation represented a very different process from the norm, in that clients were the 'givers'; I as interviewer was the recipient. Being interviewed seemed to be a novel, but welcome, experience for all of them, and the 'interesting person' status it conferred encouraged many of them to share with me the benefit of their longer life experience. One client explored the double meaning of his great age, frailty but also venerability, and recalled how he had once given up a much-desired job opportunity to care for his mother – and was now himself cared for by his daughter. He knew the cost of caring:

> *We all rely on one another, you know... Everyone, everybody,*
> *he thinks he doesn't. He thinks he can manage with the car.*
> *But you've got to rely on people.*

This is such simple advice that it seems a truism, and therefore easily disregarded. Yet it was said from a place of experience – experience beyond that of clinical staff, managers or even relatives. This is the place in which people with dementia exist, and it follows that great attention should be paid to everything that can be ascertained about that place.

What happens when an elderly person with dementia *is* included in the care process? There was one client whose wife had insisted that his condition always be openly discussed with him: that is, his awareness was recognised and he was involved in decision making. I interviewed him on the first day of his return to the unit after suffering a stroke. Although shaken by the experience, he remained optimistic in his outlook, and clearly voiced what was to him the key issue: interdependence.

I've been in places where you think to yourself: 'Well, I'm finished. Don't know what to do, don't know where to start!' And all that. Then something pops up – could be only a tu' penny-ha'penny little thing, but you feel as though – it feels really that you've got a prop there really but you can't see the prop.

'The prop', he went on to explain, was the help and support of other people. He referred fondly to the staff as 'teenagers' (acknowledging the age difference) and went on to say what he valued most in the unit:

I love it here...because it's an anchorage... You know, not because you've got to lean completely on it, I'm not leaning on nobody, but you know there's somebody there if you want it. Because we all think really that we're so self-satisfied or what-have-you that we can do it all ourselves. But we can't – no we can't.

He put in a plea for the recognition that most people have something to offer:

Most people, you know, I expect you find, are so bright. People are brighter than we think...give them half a chance, they can be resourceful, they can be helpful... You don't have to bend down on people, not that at all, no. It's give and take. Yes, I love that – give and take.

There was also the client who was always anxious to be 'helping' the staff, seeing cookery groups in this light. A busy family woman all her life, she expressed her sense of isolation now that people didn't seem to want to visit her anymore, but most of all she regretted that she was no longer needed. Another client interviewed during one of his periods of 'respite care', told of how he dreaded coming in because he had nightmares; but he knew his wife 'needed rest'. And several of the staff interviewed remarked on how concerned for their carers clients often were. In other words, care as consideration and concern already flows *from* clients as well as towards them. The construction of *dependence* occurs when care is only allowed to flow in one direction; and when care is a one-way street it is always an exercise of power, no matter how well-intentioned. When awareness and concern are mutually recognised, then care can be a two-way street – to the benefit of all involved.

Organisational characteristics determine care practice

I found that everyone involved needed to be cared for, and to have their 'awareness' or experience recognised. The feelings associated with dependence expressed by clients showed the high emotional and psychological costs of receiving care.

But a heavy psychological and emotional price was also paid by staff and managers. To spend each working day face-to-face with the emotional pain and desperation of elderly clients with dementia could be a draining experience of disempowerment and despair. To manage such services, often with little understanding of the needs of the client group, but squeezed between diminishing resources on the one hand and the clamour of over-stressed staff on the other, could equally be a recipe for cynicism and despair. And carers spoke of how they were separated from their client-relative by a gulf of misperception, often alienated from the life of the community around them, and too desperately grateful for whatever service is provided to feel able and free to voice honestly their concerns.

Many of the individual staff, managers and family carers also admitted to feeling, in their different ways, disregarded and marginalised by others. Staff felt that managers took little account of their experience and perspectives; managers that they could not trespass into clinical territory; and carers were afraid to voice suggestions or criticisms for fear of rocking the boat that held their loved one.

A culture characterised by the trickle-down practice of disregard allows clients' experience and concerns also to be sidelined, and thus the care relationship is not only a one-way street, but also it is uninformed by the most crucial input: the clients' own concerns. So the emotional cost could be high but the effectiveness for the most handicapped low. Insofar as dependence undermines the recipient, it is inherently alien to good quality caring. A two-way street of care would be characterised by mutual recognition of the awareness and experience of all involved, including clients, and by developing the listening skills of those *without* dementia so that communication can flow both ways. Effective care for elderly people with dementia will require care organisations with a genuinely cooperative ethos, and in which companionship is the model of care practice.

References

Barnett E (1996) I need to be me! A thematic evaluation of dementia care facility based on the client perspective. Unpublished PhD thesis, University of Bath.

Jacques A (1988) *Understanding Dementia*. Edinburgh: Churchill Livingstone.

Kitwood T and Bredin K (1994) *Evaluating Dementia Care: The Dementia Care Mapping Method*. Bradford University Dementia Group (now sixth edition 1994).

Sutton L (1993) The Psychology of Memory and Meaning: a revision for re-orientation to elderly mental health. Unpublished article – personal communication with the author.

2 In sickness and in health: remembering the relationship in family caregiving for people with dementia

Charlotte L Clarke

> *I don't feel like that I want him to go on holiday (respite care).*
> *I feel like I want him to be in the house, 'cause sometimes*
> *he's good company you know, he makes you laugh.*
> *One time he made me cry a lot but now, I'm getting used*
> *to him altogether now.*
>
> Mrs N, caring for her husband

This chapter argues for greater acknowledgment of the continuing relationship between the person with dementia and their carer. However, dementia care in contemporary industrialised society may be characterised by a lack of recognition of the person who has dementia (Kitwood and Bredin, 1992) and by implication a consequent dismissal of the relationship between the individual and their family carer. Indeed, this relationship is widely abused in social policies and health care interventions. Twigg (1989a) argues that family carers have an ambiguous relationship with services who either ignore them (Pitkeathley, 1989) or exploit them (Nolan and Grant, 1989). Only recently have policies explicitly recognised the part which carers play, and in doing so they emphasise the needs which carers have, thus potentially rendering them another form of 'patient' or 'client' who requires to be cared for (UK Deptartment of Health, 1989; Carers (Recognition and Services) Act 1995).

Much research has focused on identifying the stresses and burdens faced by carers (for example Zarit et al, 1985; Chenoweth and Spencer, 1986). Consequently family caregiving has often been characterised as problematic and undesirable. However, Opie (1992) argues that 'stress is embedded in caring and not an outcome of it' and some work does recognise the positive aspects of family caregiving (Motenko, 1989; Nolan et al, 1990).

Using normalisation in caregiving

Emerging from the data analysis of research which sought an understanding of the meanings of caregiving for people with dementia (Clarke, 1995) was a theory of normalisation. Not the functionalist or materialist definition of normalisation known of in the fields of learning disability and mental health (for example Gilbert, 1993), but an interactionist definition in which family carers define, and continually redefine, their life with the person with dementia as normal. The emphasis is not on the individual but on the relationship between the person with dementia and their family carer; it is not on socially or professionally defined norms but on that which is normal to that caregiving situation at that particular point in time. The normal refers to the present relationship, and the present personality of the person who has dementia. It does not refer explicitly to the future or to any generalised normality.

However, normalisation is not easy to achieve. It is an ever-changing state of hanging onto the known (the known person and known relationship) while everything that used to make sense in a relationship ceases to do so. Normalisation, however, does offer a way of understanding chronic illness and family caregiving which, as Robinson (1993) describes, is 'clearly contradictory to the story of deviance, difficulty, and despair'. The person with dementia is not passive in normalisation. Their reciprocal actions towards the family carer (in the past as well as currently) are crucial determinants of the carers ability to normalise. Nolan et al (1995) also call for research in which reciprocity within the caregiving relationship is perceived as underpinning that care.

External validation of normality rarely occurs for people with dementia and their carers. Health and social care intervention may allow caregiving to continue but it can also emphasise the abnormal (also found by Knafl and Deatrick, 1986, in relation to children with chronic illness). For example, Mr O (who cared for his mother) felt that attending a carers' support group would merely emphasise his role as a caregiver. Health and social care professionals may have a major and frequently negative impact on normalisation, attending to illness rather than life (Robinson, 1993). The work undertaken by family carers in normalisation frequently remains unacknowledged and may even be undermined by professional carers (Clarke, 1995).

Professional practice and normalisation

The tensions between the practice of professional carers and the normalising actions of family carers need to be made explicit if there is to be any impact on the practice of professionals. These tensions fall into three areas: time, person and problem. Professional carers are largely orientated to future events, emphasising the problematic prognosis of the person with dementia and in turn devaluing the dementing person as a person. Family carers know of the past person who happens to have dementia and interpret their future in relation to that knowledge, seeking to value the individual and minimise the intrusiveness of the dementia.

That family carers have a past, which included the person with dementia, is one of the reasons that caregiving is commenced. This past life allows them access to information and a knowledge of the individual before they were ill. Their awareness of the present individual is rooted in this knowledge and it allows them to develop ties of friendship, kinship and love. Professional carers are normally denied this knowledge. They have no past with the person with dementia, no ties with a person who once did not have dementia. Their experiences commence in the present. Their knowledge lies in an awareness of others who have had dementia, others who have progressed through the course of the illness. They are therefore denied the opportunity to relate to the person with dementia as they once were, but may instead relate to the dementing person as someone facing continual decline and cognitive disability.

The need to personalise the care of people with dementia is appreciated by professional carers, but they have to achieve this without a knowledge of the pre-dementing individual. Frequently, the actions of the professional carers are determined by the primacy of treatment or assessment. For example, the professional carers' involvement with Mr N was dominated by his perceived need for safe containment. In another example, Ms Y allowed her father to regularly wander out of the house because she felt that he needed that sense of freedom and self-determination.

There are, then, two knowledge bases in action. The family carer's knowledge of the person, and the professional carer's knowledge of the illness. These knowledge bases are not held exclusively and, to some extent, attempts are made to learn of each other's knowledge. Although at times these knowledges may be in conflict, they each guide the practice of that carer.

Within normalisation, even when the person with dementia requires care beyond the knowledge and ability of the family carer, a 'normal' life is not relinquished. Their life together is redefined into another normality which embraces the difficulties surrounding someone suffering from dementia, and may also have to embrace the presence of professional carers. Mr M, for example, sees no reason why his mother's confusion and incontinence should preclude her from involvement in their financial affairs, or deny her the opportunity to go out on day trips. This contrasts with the perspective of professional carers whose purpose it is to 'assess' and, in doing so, seek out the abnormal in the individual. Thus the lives of the person with dementia and their family carer become relatively problem-orientated, dominated by what is wrong in their lives rather than what is ordinary and normal.

Professional practice within the caregiving relationship

One central concern in caring for someone with dementia is the maintenance of that person as a person. Several papers, as well as the study by the author (Clarke, 1995), bear testimony to the difficulties of achieving this. Kitwood (1990, p195) writes that:

> *From the standpoint of the 'standard paradigm' (of relentless nervous tissue degeneration) there is a disease process in the brain of someone who, as a person, remains unknown and irrelevant. Vaguely, on the margins, there is the question of biography and life-setting.*

For family carers, it is the dementia which is in the margin. The person remains entirely and wholly relevant to the relationship between the person with dementia and their family carer.

The challenge for professional practice is to make this paradigm shift, to grasp the dementing person as a person and to support the family carer in their quest to hang onto the interpersonal aspects of living with someone with a cognitive loss, a need also acknowledged by Kitson (1987) and Orona (1990). To achieve this may mean changing some aspects of current practice. There is a need to question the use of health care interventions which reinforce the abnormality of caregiving and the pathology of dementia. For example, the appropriateness of respite and day care for carer relief has been regularly questioned (Twigg, 1989b; Nolan and Grant, 1992).

Since any relationship exists as an interactive process, and is never a static state, that interaction between the person with dementia and the family carer can and should be acknowledged. Family carers function within this relationship, and its interactive process profoundly affects their actions. For example, family carers may be reluctant to let others know of the individual's failing cognitive ability, protecting them from the social reaction of stigma, but also denying themselves and the person with dementia access to health and social care. Mrs F, for example, described the pre-diagnosis phase as 'a traumatic experience' because she was torn between accessing help and being loyal to her husband with dementia who 'didn't want people to think he was an idiot'. The wishes of the person with dementia may be a key determinant in the acceptance or refusal of service intervention by the family carer. The nature of the relationship between the person with dementia and family carer, be it reciprocal or antagonistic, was found to be a central factor in the ability to normalise a relationship (Clarke, 1995). The interdependence of the person with dementia and family carer is demonstrated by Mrs P, caring for her husband, who felt she would 'not last long after he's gone', a situation also found by Orona (1990).

The dominant professional approach to dementia care, emphasising the abnormal, the pathological and the prognosis of relentless deterioration, undermines the relationship-orientated approach to caregiving. It does, however, offer structure and some meaning to events and allows planning to be made for future problems, although arguably thereby contributing to their creation (Clarke and Keady, 1996). Normalisation, however, is grounded in the relationship of the person with dementia and the family carer, and is woven into the fabric of their lives. It operates in relation to the past, the person and the problem-free.

Family carers want, and work towards maintaining, a relationship with someone who is important to them, and in which disease and problems can be kept minimally intrusive. This may be achieved through normalisation, and for many it is achieved with little or no professional carer intervention. Where some intervention is necessary to support the caregiving relationship, that intervention will best support normalisation if it acknowledges the family carer's knowledge base as at least equal, but very different, to a professional knowledge base. An effective care intervention will make judicious use of both these knowledge bases, with the aim of retaining the dementing person as a person, and fulfilling the needs of the relationship between the family and the person with dementia. Hasselkus (1988) writes of the need for professional and family carers to recognise the context of meaning in which their expertise is embedded, and challenges carers to make these meanings accessible to each other.

As professionals we perhaps need to look to the individual's past instead of our perception of their future, to the person instead of the illness and to seeking freedom from problems instead of the problematic. In protecting a relationship against the ravages of dementia, family carers work to save a person from the worst effects of one of the most destructive diseases of our time. The challenge for health and social care is to support them in this quest.

References

Carers (Recognition and Services) Act (1995) London: HMSO.

Chenoweth B and Spencer B (1986) Dementia: the experience of family caregivers. *The Gerontologist* 26, 267-272.

Clarke CL (1995) Care of elderly people suffering from dementia and their co-resident informal carers. In Heyman B (ed) *Researching User Perspectives On Community Health Care*. London: Chapman and Hall.

Clarke CL and Keady J (1996) Researching dementia care and family caregiving: extending ethical responsibilities. *Health Care in Later Life* 1(2), 85-95.

Gilbert T (1993) Learning disability nursing: from normalisation to materialism – towards a new paradigm. *Journal of Advanced Nursing* 18, 1604-1609.

Hasselkus BR (1988) Meaning in family caregiving: perspectives on caregiver/professional relationships. *The Gerontologist* 28(5), 686-691.

Kitson AL (1987) A comparative analysis of lay-caring and professional (nursing) caring relationships. *International Journal of Nursing Studies* 24(2), 155-165.

Kitwood T (1990) The dialectics of dementia with particular reference to Alzheimer's disease. *Ageing and Society* 10, 177-196.

Kitwood T and Bredin K (1992) Towards a theory of dementia care: personhood and well-being. *Ageing and Society* 12, 269-287.

Knafl KA and Deatrick JA (1986) How families manage chronic conditions: an analysis of the concept of normalisation. *Research in Nursing and Health* 9, 215-222.

Motenko AK (1989) The frustrations, gratifications, and well-being of dementia caregivers. *The Gerontologist* 29(2), 166-172.

Nolan M and Grant G (1989) Addressing the needs of informal carers: a neglected area of nursing practice. *Journal of Advanced Nursing* 14(11), 950-962.

Nolan M, Grant G and Ellis N (1990) Stress is in the eye of the beholder: reconceptualising the measurement of carer burden. *Journal of Advanced Nursing* 15(5), 544-555.

Nolan M and Grant G (1992) Respite care: challenging tradition. *British Journal of Nursing* 1(3), 129-131.

Nolan M, Keady J and Grant G (1995) Developing a typology of family care: implications for nurses and other service providers. *Journal of Advanced Nursing* 21, 256-265.

Opie A (1992) *There's Nobody There: Community Care of Confused Older People.* Auckland: Oxford University Press.

Orona CJ (1990) Temporality and identity loss due to Alzheimer's disease. *Social Sciences and Medicine* 30(11), 1247-1256.

Pitkeathley J (1989) *It's My Duty, Isn't It? The Plight of Carers in Our Society.* London: Souvenir Press.

Robinson CA (1993) Managing life with a chronic condition: the story of normalisation. *Qualitative Health Research* 3(1), 6-28.

Twigg J (1989a) Models of carers: how do social care agencies conceptualise their relationship with informal carers? *Journal of Social Policy* 18(1), 53-66.

Twigg J (1989b) Not taking the strain. *Community Care* 77, 16-19.

UK Department of Health (1989) *Caring for People – Community Care in the Next Decade and Beyond.* London: HMSO.

Zarit SH, Orr NK and Zarit JM (1985) *The Hidden Victims of Alzheimer's Disease: Families Under Stress.* New York University Press.

3 Insight and dementia

Andrew Fairbairn

Introduction

Dementia is a progressive decline of cognitive function, and insight may be defined as the ability to understand one's own problems. Thus, taken at face value cognitive failure leads to loss of insight. However, there is an intriguing literature that suggests communication is the core problem and that quite severely demented people are capable of insight, but only problems with language make communication impossible (see Killick, 1994). It can be argued that loss of insight is a helpful protection in the more severe stages of dementia, whereas in the early stages of dementia insight maybe of value and its early loss may be a major problem. Markova and Berrios (1995) discussing the concept of insight, regard it as a construct and define it as 'self-knowledge'.

Background

McDaniel et al (1991) have shown that a decreased level of insight correlates with severity of dementia and that an increase of 31 per cent in the loss of insight was perceived in patients whose 'progress' was monitored over a period of two years.

Claims have been made that certain types of dementia are accompanied by increased loss of insight, for example frontal type dementia. Clinicians have generally subscribed to the view that vascular dementia is more likely to lead to patchy insight when compared to Alzheimer's disease, but Verhey et al (1995) studied insight and personality change in mild cases of vascular dementia, probable Alzheimer's disease and normal controls, and showed that depression, lack of insight and personality change did not favour vascular dementia over Alzheimer's disease. Lack of insight appeared to relate more to severity than to presumed aetiology.

Mangone et al (1991) have created an insight score by measuring the discrepancies between patient reports and carer reports. In addition to the correlation of loss of insight to severity, they found increased impairment associated with paranoid ideation. Neuropsychological testing in this study indicated that impaired insight appeared to have two components namely confabulation and anosognosia (a lack of concern for a particular disability) which in turn imply pre-frontal and right hemisphere dysfunction.

De Bettignies et al (1990) looked at insight in dementia and found no relation to age, educational status, mental status or level of depression, but there was a significant correlation with the degree of caregiver burden.

Loebel et al (1990) showed that preserved fluency of speech appeared to be associated with poor self-awareness of memory deficits. Weinstein et al (1994) correlated denial with age of onset, severity, course and duration of dementia. They also tried to differentiate denial, or unawareness, from the concept of loss of insight and argue that there is a lack of correlation with severity in the case of denial. In other words, denial and insight are different concepts.

Insight may be an indicator of an atypical aetiology. For example Zan et al (1994) report a case of dementia with retained insight associated with naso-pharyngeal carcinoma.

Markova and Berrios (1995) discuss a putative biological model of insight detailing the neurological and physiological processes in such a model.

Insight and information

Over the last twenty years there has been a considerable increase in knowledge about dementia in the general population. The public perception has changed from the view that dementia is an inevitable progression of old age through to an understanding of dementia as an illness. Nevertheless, many older dementia sufferers are from a cultural background where they regard memory failure, in particular, as a normal inevitability. These sufferers do not therefore expect substantial information on their diagnosis and prognosis. Would clear diagnostic information, if routinely given, assist in the retention of insight into the disease process? This is, of course, an entirely separate issue from the information that needs to be given to the carer and the subsequent insight of the carer into the disease and its progress.

Insight and cooperation

Lack of insight in dementia sufferers is probably the commonest cause of lack of cooperation within care. There is frequently tension due to the desire to protect the individual's right to freedom and the possibly paternalistic interventions of the professionals. Lack of cooperation can lead to packages of care being rejected or to a restriction in the choice of packages. For example, if an individual were aware that he was suffering from dementia then he may accept that it would reduce stress upon his spouse if he attended a day centre which he otherwise would hate doing. Conversely, the refusal to attend a day centre may lead to specialist sitter services being arranged in the house. This may show admirable flexibility of response, but it can create a problem for the spouse who is unable to relax in her own home and has to go out of the house to gain relief.

Insight and carer stress

Dementia has been described as a family illness: the whole family are affected, but it is the sufferer who is most likely to be unaware of the problems. This is stressful for the carer but the sufferer's lack of insight can further increase the stress. If the key carer is a spouse then the intricate dynamics of a lengthy relationship can add another dimension to carer stress and the issue of insight. For example, throughout a marriage the husband may have decided when his shirts were dirty but now that he is dementing he may forget to change his shirt. However, when his wife prompts him that his shirt looks dirty, his response is likely to be that he has always decided when he needed a fresh shirt. His wife is already stressed with the awareness of the illness and she becomes further stressed by his inability to recognise when assistance, which he now needs, is being given to him.

Insight, suicide and terminal care

Surprisingly, perhaps, patients in the early stages who are informed that they have a dementing illness and are able to retain information and insight, very rarely attempt suicide. However Rohde et al (1995) reported two cases, one aged 50 and the other aged 80, who did commit suicide. Both subjects were highly educated professionals in the early stages of dementia with unusually intact insight. They had been disappointed by the results of experimental drug treatment trials.

These rarities aside, the infrequency of suicide may be in part due to a lack of understanding of the potential personal indignity of the severe stages of dementia.

Increasingly people are taking control over their own terminal care and in many ways this is due to the expansion of the hospice movement. The inevitable loss of insight in the severe stages of dementia means that dementia sufferers have a loss of control over their own terminal care. This is a particularly difficult area to consider, but is it possible that loss of insight into the condition is indeed a factor in the ability of dementia sufferers to survive? Paradoxically, do they survive for longer because they are unaware of their illness?

Insight and the right to independence

Apart from the more obvious issues such as the right to refuse packages of support so, in turn, placing increasing burdens upon carers and the local community, there is a certain point where a varying degree of insight may be the crucial factor in the right to remain independent. This may be hard to separate from personality factors, but there is often a difficult judgement involved as to whether to allow dementia sufferers to live without dignity and at risk for a shorter period of time rather than to be institutionalised, kept clean and smart, and probably survive for longer. The difficult judgement for professionals is often one of what the individual, had he/she reasonable insight, would have wanted in these circumstances? The other element concerning the right to independence is that all human beings live in some form of society with the concomitant responsibilities to that society. Therefore, there may be some limit that society is entitled to place upon that individual, whether the individual is insightful or not.

Insight and legal interventions

It is not the purpose of this chapter to discuss in any great depth the medico-legal aspects of dementia. However, dementia is a mental illness and so is covered by Mental Health Act legislation. Difficult decisions about compulsory admission or guardianship for dementia sufferers will often crucially pivot on the sufferer's insight into the condition. Similarly, advance directives, such as enduring power of attorney and other pieces of legislation relating to the management of personal affairs, all tacitly acknowledge that insight, or more accurately the lack of insight, is a crucial element in any formal implementation; yet legislation does not explicitly use the term 'insight'.

Car driving is often seen as problematic. However, Rees et al (1995) reported that about 50 per cent of demented drivers who were advised to stop did so, often following carer advice. In most instances carer insight into the driving problems was good.

Can insight be induced?

Is it possible with a condition such as dementia, which involves the failure to retain information, that insight can be induced sensitively, appropriately and helpfully? In the field of functional psychosis, schizophrenia in particular, Kemp and David (1995) have discussed psycho-educational and behavioural family therapy approaches that appear to improve insight. Of course, there must be uncertainty as to whether approaches that could be applied in functional psychosis can be applied in a progressive organic psychosis. For example, does repeated correct information, as used in the techniques of reality/orientation, induce some form of insight? If the loss of insight is one of the few protections in this terrible illness, is it appropriate to try and improve insight, presumably for the purpose of allowing the tidying-up of a personal life and the opportunity to sort out personal affairs?

The future

Insight and the lack of insight is a crucial ingredient in the progressive disorder that is dementia. Problems relating to insight are everyday issues for carers and professionals dealing with dementia sufferers, yet little attempt has been made to analyse the meaning of insight, the consequences of this or to consider the implications in relation to information, prognosis management and consent.

A concerted, multidisciplinary research programme is now required to look at:

• biological markers of insight in dementia;
• premorbid personality factors and insight in dementia;
• the value of educational and other training programmes;
• ethical and legal dilemmas in relation to insight and dementia;
• informed consent in research studies in relation to insight in dementia;
• insight as a factor in carer stress;
• insight as a variable in the delivery of care packages;
• insight as a factor in the natural history of the dementias.

References

DeBettignies BH, Mahurin RK and Pirozzolo FJ (1990) Insight for impairment in independent living skills in Alzheimer's Disease and multi-infarct dementia. *Journal of Clinical and Experimental Neuropsychology* 12(2), 355-363.

Kemp R and David A (1995) Psychosis: insight and compliance. *Current Opinion in Psychiatry* 8(6), 357-361.

Killick J (1994) *Please Give Me Back My Personality!* Stirling: Dementia Services Development Centre.

Loebel JP, Dager SR, Berg G and Hyde TS (1990) Fluency of speech and self awareness of memory deficit in Alzheimer's Disease. *International Journal of Geriatric Psychiatry* 5(1), 41-45.

Mangone CA, Hier DB, Gorelick PB, Ganellen RJ et al (1991) Impaired insight in Alzheimer's Disease. *Journal of Geriatric Psychiatry and Neurology* 4(4), 189-193.

Markova A and Berrios G (1995) Insight in Psychiatry. *Journal of Nervous and Mental Disease* 183(12), 743-751.

McDaniel KD, Edland SD and Heyman A (1995) The relationship between level of insight and severity of dementia in Alzheimer's Disease. *Alzheimer's Disease and Associated Disorders* 9(2), 101-104.

Rees J, Gayer A and Phillips G (1995) Assessment and management of the dementing driver. *Journal of Mental Health* 4(2), 165-176.

Rohde K, Peskind ER and Raskind MA (1995) Suicide in two patients with Alzheimer's Disease. *Journal of the American Geriatrics Society* 43(2), 187-189.

Weinstein EA, Friedland RP and Wagner EE (1994) Denial/unawareness of impairment and symbolic behaviour in Alzheimer's Disease. *Neuropsychiatry, Neuropsychology and Behavioural Neurology* 7(3), 176-184.

Verhey FRJ, Ponds RWMM, Rozendaal N and Jolles J (1995) Depression, insight and personality change in Alzheimer's Disease and vascular dementia. *Journal of Geriatric Psychiatry and Neurology* 8(1), 23-27.

Zan MDA, Varma SL, Sellandurai BM, Sharma HS et al (1994) Dementia associated with nasopharyngeal carcinoma. *European Psychiatry* 9(1), 53-54.

4 Between a rock and a hard place: the impact of dementia on young carers

Jane Gilliard

Why should dementia be an issue for children and young people? It is, after all, a condition which mostly affects older people. Indeed we know that age is a risk factor for developing dementia. It profoundly affects the person at the centre, the person experiencing the dementia. But in addition, it impacts on all those who have any contact with the person with dementia, especially the caregivers. As a rough guide, two-thirds of carers are spouses and are therefore likely to be older people themselves; of the remaining one-third, most are daughters and daughters-in-law, and are most likely to be in mid-life. These are the main carers. There are also secondary carers – those who support the main carer – and then there are significant others who are affected because a family member has dementia, or because they work with people with dementia.

Traditionally we have focused our concern on the principal caregiver, considering service provision to give them space and to support them. But we should also pay attention to the needs of all those affected, and this may well include a number of young people whose lives are affected by having a relative who has dementia, usually a grandparent. For example:

> *Clare is 12, her brother, Mark, is 10 and her sister, Marie, is 7. Their grandmother comes originally from Eastern Europe, but has lived in this country for fifty years. She has dementia, and is no longer able to communicate in English, having reverted to her first language. When the time came that she could no longer live alone, it was impossible to find a suitable placement for her because of the*

difficulties of communication. She moved in with her son and his
family. Marie gave up her bedroom and moved in with Clare.

Clare bitterly resents this intrusion into her privacy, just at a time when she particularly wants some personal space. She wants to be able to put up pictures of her idols on the walls, play her records at full volume and entertain her friends in her room. But now she has to share this room with her little sister. This leads to arguments between the sisters. It also makes Clare feel resentful towards her brother who has still got his own room, and towards her grandmother who is, in Clare's eyes, the cause of all her problems.

For Clare's parents there is now the added strain of having an ageing parent with dementia to live with them, and the internal family friction which this has caused. What was a happy family unit has become a source for arguments. Clare has turned almost overnight from being a happy young girl into a touchy, argumentative adolescent.

For some families there is very serious concern caused by the behaviour of the person with dementia, as in the case of Susie:

Susie is 14, her sister, Kate, is 12. Their grandmother has always
lived with them and now she has dementia. Susie's and Kate's
mother works part-time. Her mother (the girls' grandmother) has
always been in the habit of preparing lunch for her daughter's
return from work. But as her dementia progresses, it's becoming
harder for her to manage to lay the table and prepare the food.
One day during the school holidays, Susie decided it would be easier
if she prepared lunch for her mother and began to lay the table.
Her grandmother became extremely agitated about this, picked up a
knife and tried to attack Susie with it.

Susie and Kate became frightened of their grandmother and could no longer be left alone in the house with her. The Social Services child protection team felt that there was a significant risk in this family. They recommended that grandmother should be admitted to residential care. The family were set against this as the grandmother had always lived with them. Eventually the authorities decided that the risk was such that either grandmother was admitted to residential care or the girls would have to be received into care. The grandmother went into a local residential home.

For most young people, the relative with dementia will be a grandparent. But for some, it will be their own parent and, with the changes that are occurring in our modern society, perhaps they will increasingly live within one parent families, like Laura and Alex:

> *Laura is 19. She left school after taking her GCSEs and worked as a companion for an elderly man, before taking up her present post as a care assistant at a local home for older people. She is engaged to Robert and they would like to get their own flat and move in together. She enjoys going to the disco or out for a drink with Robert. She is very keen on rock music, and particularly the local rock scene.*

> *Alex is 15 years old. He will be taking nine GCSEs in the summer and hopes to go to the local sixth form college to study for his A levels. He plays football for the school team, enjoys mountain biking, and has a wide circle of friends including a girlfriend. Laura and Alex have been brought up in a single parent household since their mother died five years ago, and they have recently learnt that their father has dementia, probably Alzheimer's disease.*

Alex sometimes finds it difficult to settle to do his homework. There isn't anyone at home to drive him on – he has to be solely responsible for himself. The temptation to rush work or miss it altogether is very strong. Sometimes his father is wandering round the house making a lot of noise and it's hard to find the space in which to work and revise. Sometimes his father wanders into Alex's room and moves all his papers or rearranges them so when Alex returns they are out of order. Alex has to be responsible for getting himself up and off to school on time in the morning. He resents any attempt at discipline by Laura – she is, after all, only his big sister, so who does she think she is?

Alex's wide circle of friends often meet in each other's homes. They used to come to Alex's home, but his father would often say or do very bizarre things. Alex tried for a long time to hide his father's problems from his friends. He didn't want to stand out amongst his friends as being the odd one – the one with a 'loony Dad'. When he could no longer hide the problems, he tried to explain to his friends. Some of them were quite understanding at first, but for most of them dementia was something well beyond their normal experience. They stopped meeting at Alex's house or calling for him. Alex became more and more isolated, and increasingly angry – with his mother because she had died and left them, and with his father because he was no longer a proper father. Sometimes he would shout at his father, 'Why can't you be a normal Dad, like other people's?'

The staff at Alex's school were anxious to have someone with whom they could liaise about his behaviour and work. Alex needed someone to represent him at parent's evenings, when his work and plans for the future could be discussed. On a personal level, the rest of the football squad have someone standing on the touchline shouting for them – Alex has nobody.

Laura found herself missing days at work because the responsibility for caring for their father fell on her shoulders more and more. She had sleepless nights when her father wandered round the house, and then she felt too tired to go to work. She spent so much energy caring for her father, that it was difficult to summon up more energies to care for the older people in the home. Eventually she decided to give up work and become her father's full-time carer. This meant that she had less income, and that she was at home far more, and she found this harder than she'd imagined that she would.

All these young people need a variety of special support, as well as sharing some of the needs of any other carer. They need and deserve information about dementia, its progress and prognosis, but this information should be pitched at their own level so that they can understand in their own way what is happening. They need befriending. All carers say that caring is a lonely task – how much more so when you're coping with growing up at the same time. Clare needs someone who will listen when she wants to talk about how unfair it all feels now that her grandmother has come to live with them. The issue for service providers is who should provide this support – a social worker from the children's team who has little or no working knowledge of dementia, or someone from the elderly care team who has no current experience of working with children and young people?

Young people need advice about their entitlements. Laura should have been informed about the Invalid Care Allowance when she gave up work to look after her father so that she could receive the maximum money to which she is entitled. Young people also need advice about the services available to help them and the person with dementia. At present these are very limited. There are less than forty young carers schemes across the country, and similarly few services for people with early onset dementia. But it's worth talking about what is available. Laura decided to go to a support group for people who care for someone with dementia. She's about forty years younger than the next youngest carer, but she finds it extremely helpful to listen to others, to exchange feelings and stories, and has found it a safe haven in which she can cry and let go of some of her feelings about what's happened to her family.

Young people need an advocate. Alex deserves someone to be his representative at those events to which parents normally go – parents evening, football matches and interviews for college.

As well as support for those young people who are directly affected by having a family member or friend who has dementia, all young people need to be informed and educated about dementia. The words 'dementia' and

'Alzheimer's disease' still carry a stigma which makes it hard for carers to explain the condition to others and which increases their sense of isolation. If we can break down the barriers by educating young people about dementia, then the public of tomorrow will be better informed and the people with dementia of tomorrow and their carers (and this will undoubtedly include you and me) will be part of a more caring and understanding society.

Note

The case studies used in this article are drawn from Jane's experience of working as a counsellor with carers of people with dementia. Names have been changed to protect the identity of the families.

References

Evans E *It's Me, Grandma, It's Me*. Available from the Alzheimer's Disease Society, Gordon House, 10 Greencoat Place, London SW1P 1PH.

Gilliard J (1995) *The Long and Winding Road: A Young Person's Guide to Dementia*. Petersfield: Wrightson BioMedical Publishing.

5 Hearing the voice of people with dementia

Malcolm Goldsmith

When people want to know about dementia, to whom do they turn? Or, more specifically, whose voice do they listen to? In my experience it is to the voice of the medical profession. The results of their inquiries can vary a great degree, dependent upon the knowledge and skill of the medical opinion. Failing that, to whom do they turn? Probably to any other kind of 'expert', perhaps a social worker or some other form of service provider. Over the last decade we have witnessed the appearance of another voice, that of the carer. At long last it is being recognised that the men and women who care for people with dementia day in and day out may have a contribution to make, and may have insight and information which can open up the world of dementia to the inquirer. And there the matter has rested – until recently.

It is as though there is a vast invisible pyramid. At the top are the medical experts, and below them other medics who may not be quite so expert, and below them the experts from other fields, and then others who are not quite such experts, and down at the bottom, with a very broad base, are the hundreds of thousands of carers. But there is another level, one which has largely been ignored until recently, and that is the level inhabited by the people who have dementia. What about their voice? Who hears that?

The prevailing wisdom seems to be that the very nature of the illnesses, which are at the heart of dementia, means that the people so affected are unable to reflect on or communicate their feelings and views on their situation. That view is now being questioned.

Behind the questioning lies an enormous philosophical issue. What is the nature of the person with dementia? Does the illness rob the person of the very essence of what it means to be a person, are they, in fact, in the process of 'unbecoming', as some people have argued? Or is the person still essentially there, as a person, but limited and handicapped by the nature of their illness? Asking questions about the essence of the person only serves to highlight just how little we actually know about the nature of dementia. We do not know, for instance, if the memory itself has been lost or if it is the access to the memory which has been lost. If it is the memory itself, then how do we account for those occasional moments of lucidity which may appear even when the illness has reached an advanced state?

In recent years there have been a number of studies with people with dementia which demonstrate that it is actually possible to ascertain their views about the services which they receive. Work done in the United States (Yale, 1993) and elsewhere has shown that it is possible for people with dementia to share their hopes and fears about their condition with other people in a similar situation and with skilled counsellors. Valerie Sinason (1992) has written a very moving account of a year long process of psychotherapy with one person with dementia, and Heidi Hamilton (1994) has traced a pattern of communication with someone over a period of four and a half years. There are also one or two accounts of what it is like to have dementia written by the people themselves (Davis, 1989; McGowin, 1993), and more and more of these accounts are now coming into the public domain. There is little doubt in my mind that people with dementia are able to express their views to a much greater degree and for a longer period of time than has generally been thought to be possible. But this is not to say that the process is easy, nor that it is always possible.

First, there must be a belief that communication is possible. Without such a belief, or a commitment to explore such a belief, then we are unlikely to identify the clues which might come our way. Second, there must be a willingness to respect the time and pace of the person with dementia. Communication may not be possible on Monday morning, but may be possible on Thursday evening! Communication cannot be rushed and we need endless patience and tolerance. Third, we have to explore the world of metaphor and symbolism, and recognise that we have to approach language construction with a fresh set of suppositions and expectations. Fourth, we have to be open to possibilities for non-verbal communication, and we need to take on board the suggestion that so called 'challenging behaviour' is, itself, an attempt to communicate. Finally, we must always honour the person, and determining what 'honour' might mean in any particular set of circumstances may itself be quite a task.

The responsibility for easing the communication process must be ours. It is a skilled job and we will need a great deal of patience. Perhaps we should approach it as though learning a foreign language – some people seem to be naturally gifted and born linguists and a new language seems to come easily to them, but *everyone* has to work at it. It requires effort, commitment, skill and a natural aptitude. And there are few better ways of learning a language than using it within the appropriate context.

Similarly, when we are with people with dementia, to hear their voice may be quite a challenge. It may tax us intellectually and stretch our imagination; it will test our patience and it will bring surprises and setbacks but also moments of clarity which make it all worthwhile.

Let me close with a word of warning. If it is true that many people think that people with dementia cannot express an opinion, it is also true that some people assume too quickly that they know just what it is that the person wishes to communicate. There is always the danger that people with dementia respond to carers by saying or doing what they perceive is wanted from them. The more severe the disability, the more dependent the person is upon other people's views of their needs, and the more vulnerable they are to low expectations.

Hearing the voice of people with dementia is both a challenge and a journey, and we ourselves will be affected in the process. Many people prefer not to take up that challenge and convince themselves that not only is there no voice, but basically that there is no real person there either. As the illness progresses it often becomes more and more difficult to hold on to the conviction that there is still a real, living sentient being within the body that is before us. We still do not know enough about the nature of 'being' to dismiss such a conviction, and while the jury is still out on this matter it is surely good practice to work on the assumption that there still is a person in there, however difficult we find that to accept.

I actually believe that there is, and also that there is still a voice, or rather, I work on the assumption that there is until it is proved otherwise. How we hear that voice and how we encourage and interpret it must surely be one of the next areas to be addressed in our research and training programmes.

References

Davis R (1989) *My Journey into Alzheimer's Disease*. Amersham: Scripture Press.

Goldsmith M (1996) *Hearing the Voice of People with Dementia*. London: Jessica Kingsley.

Hamilton HE (1994) *Conversations with an Alzheimer's Patient*. Cambridge: Cambridge University Press.

McGowin D (1993) *Living in the Labyrinth: A Personal Journey Through the Maze of Alzheimer's*. San Francisco: Elder Books.

Sinason V (1992) *Mental Handicap and the Human Condition: New approaches from the Tavistock*. London: Free Association Books.

Yale R (1993) *A Guide to Facilitating Support Groups for Newly Diagnosed Alzheimer's Patients*. This monograph and various others which are related are obtainable from LCS 1067 Filbert Street, Suite 100, San Francisco, California 94133, USA.

6 Maintaining involvement: a meta concept to describe the dynamics of dementia

John Keady

Introduction

Recent studies, which have attempted to interpret the needs of people with the first signs of dementia, have all commented upon the past failure of research inquiry and service provision to address fully this population group (see for example, Froggatt, 1988; Gillies, 1995; Keady and Nolan, 1995 a,b; Goldsmith, 1996). Indeed, qualitative studies which have attempted a social construction of the experience of dementia have usually been centred on the family carer (Wilson, 1989 a,b; Taraborelli, 1993; Askham, 1995) or on interpreting the continuum of cognitive and behavioural coping efforts displayed by this group (Bowers, 1987; Clarke, 1995; Harvath, 1994). To date there has only been limited attention paid to the development of a social construction of dementia either from an individual perspective (Gubrium, 1987; Sabat and Harré, 1992) or from the meanings that this jointly holds to the individual and family members concerned (Keady and Nolan, 1994; Wuest et al, 1994; LeNavenec, 1995).

Study methodology

To address further this area of need, a grounded theory study (Glaser and Strauss, 1967) was conducted by the author between 1992 and 1995. The study involved in-depth interviews with 58 carers of people with dementia and 11 interviews with people experiencing the first signs of dementia. The study methodology and ethical implications of conducting research interviews on sensitive topics has been described more fully elsewhere (Keady and Nolan, 1994; 1995 a,b,c; 1996; Clarke and Keady, 1996).

The first signs of dementia

By adopting this approach a new basic social process emerged from the data which linked the myriad of experiences exhibited by people with dementia, and their family carers, throughout its duration, that is from the time of symptom onset through to the carers' adjustment at the end of caring. This basic social process, or meta concept, has been termed 'maintaining involvement' and its properties were seen to move in time, purpose and meaning. Moreover, 'maintaining involvement' also underpinned personal adjustment and coping behaviours and moved across, and within, relationships, support networks and professional interventions. A practical illustration of this social process follows.

Maintaining involvement by taking the initiative
In an effort to maintain involvement during the impact of dementia, individuals underwent a transition through three dimensions:
- taking the initiative;
- responding to events;
- withdrawing from situations.

This process is displayed graphically in Figure 6.1.

Figure 6.1 The experience of dementia: transitional dimensions

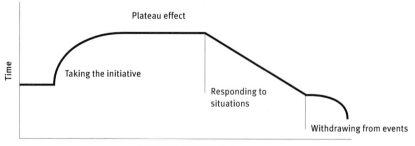

The first of these dimensions has been termed 'taking the initiative'. Taking the initiative describes the active adjustment and coping responses at the onset of dementia, and which are used by the individual to manage the impact of new sensory experiences. Drawing on the interview data these new sensory experiences took a number of forms including:

First noticed signs of dementia
- problem-solving difficulties;
- being unable to concentrate for prolonged periods;
- inability to immediately put names to faces;
- quickly loosing track of conversations;
- feeling disassociated from reality;
- becoming sad and depressed;
- feeling unduly angry;
- tearfulness;
- feeling and becoming lost in familiar surroundings;
- not being able to coordinate fully and control speech and action;
- writing block;
- heightened sense of taste and smell.

Note: This list is not intended to represent fully all reported first signs. Some people reported an initial experience of a combination of such signs

Interestingly, however, no one person in this study translated these first signs to the onset of dementia, and the decision making process which led to this outcome involved the following pattern:

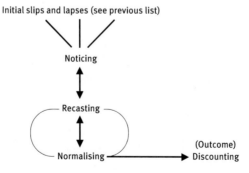

Initially, this decision making process operates at an intuitive level. The person experiencing these initial slips and lapses was aware that something was wrong, but they were unable to translate this into any meaningful context. In other words, the first sign(s) were noticed, recast (thought about), normalised (its probably due to age/stress/retirement) and then discounted (it isn't anything to be worried about). However, over time, repeated and accumulated exposure to such slips and lapses heightened the noticing and recasting processes, and facilitated the entry of both suspecting and acting into the decision making cycle. This new and active phase is conceptualised as follows:

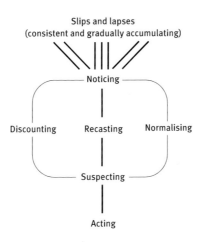

For the individual concerned it became vitally important to act upon the suspicions that something was quite seriously wrong and it is usually at this point where *deliberate* action was taken to preserve the self. This was achieved by deploying the tactic of 'closing down' in order to 'construct a new me' from within a cumulative experience of loss. The tactic of closing down emerged as being private and secretive in nature, and was extremely distressing for those close to the individual as they remained completely in the dark over its real purpose and function. One of the most compelling features of this transition was the need to keep the initial signs hidden and secret. Indeed, it is important to emphasise that this desire was all embracing and not openly communicated even in relationships which were obviously very loving and close.

The following quotation from the study, provided by a 67 year old man with Alzheimer's disease, attempts to illustrate the secretive nature of this behaviour and, for the person concerned, their heightened feelings of tension and anxiety:

I knew something was wrong with me, but I didn't want this to be seen by anyone else. I wanted to stay 'normal' but I found it was (long pause) hard. A struggle. (pause) I had to make lots of lists and keep them in the house or car. We argued a lot because I never wanted to go out. Scared you see. I was always terrified my wife would find out.

However, despite this recognition, there remained a diminishing hope that things 'would get back to normal', and this was also expressed during interviews when the diagnosis of dementia was known – hence the loose links back to 'normalising' and 'discounting' represented in the previous diagram. There also remained a continuing need for 'Keeping It All Hidden' and, by employing this strategy, it allowed the person with (unconfined) dementia the opportunity for 'maintaining involvement' within their newly found reality. To support this process the development, maintenance and shaping of routines appeared of crucial importance to the individual with the first signs of dementia (Keady and Nolan, 1995 a,b). Furthermore, the person began to construct a range of expert behaviours in managing their own shifting reality, a behaviour illustrated on Figure 6.1 during the relative stability of the 'Plateau Effect', before others gradually begin to notice that all may not be right – thus for family members, and/or work colleagues, commencing once again the intuitive decision making process, involving noticing – recasting – normalising – discounting.

Practice implications

By taking this approach one step further a social construction of the experience of dementia can begin to emerge. This final diagram attempts to illustrate the strategy of 'Keeping It All Hidden' and the personal tactics that are necessary for maintaining involvement in this process.

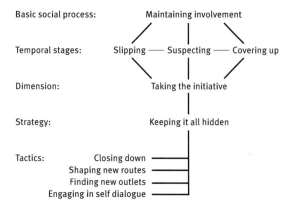

It was surprising how often the tactic of 'engaging in self-dialogue' emerged and acted as a safety valve for people with the first signs of dementia who wanted to verbally reassure themselves that they were 'doing okay'. In effect, these behaviours and actions served to protect people with dementia and, later, their family supporters from its full impact. Interestingly, these strategies were later selectively used by the carer once the individual began to respond to events, and not to actively shape them.

Conclusion

In the author's opinion, the development of services to people with the first signs of dementia will emerge as a major issue for health and social care providers in the next decade and beyond. Provision of memory training and support groups for people with the first signs of dementia is gaining a momentum in the USA (Yale, 1996) and, within the UK, the Alzheimer's Disease Society has placed an increasing emphasis on the need for early diagnosis and the provision of sensitive and tailored information (ADS, 1996). However, to begin to build upon these advances, a comprehensive educational strategy for practitioner training is necessary coupled to a health education campaign on recognising the first signs of dementia. At present such approaches remain in their infancy and much remains to be done. However, the prospect for advancing dementia care practice in these arenas must not be lost, and neither should the opportunity to construct interventions on the basis of its perceived meanings to the individual concerned.

References

Alzheimer's Disease Society (1996) *I'm told I have dementia*. Information booklet, London: ADS.

Askham J (1995) Making sense of dementia: carers' perceptions. *Ageing and Society* 15, 103-114.

Bowers BJ (1987) Inter-generational caregiving: adult caregivers and their ageing parents. *Advances in Nursing Science* 9(2), 20-31.

Clarke CL (1995) Care of elderly people suffering from dementia and their co-resident informal carers. In Heyman B (ed) *Researching User Perspectives on Community Health Care*. London: Chapman and Hall, 135-149.

Clarke CL and Keady J (1996) Researching dementia care and family caregiving: extending ethical responsibilities. *Health Care in Later Life: An International Research Journal* 1(2), 87-95.

Froggatt A (1998) Self-awareness in early dementia. In Gearing B, Johnson M and Heller T (eds) *Mental Health Problems in Old Age: A Reader*. Buckingham: Open University Press, 131-136.

Gillies B (1995) *The Subjective Experience of Dementia: A Qualitative Analysis of Interviews with Dementia Sufferers and Their Carers and the Implications for Service Provision.* Stirling: Dementia Services Development Centre.

Glaser BG and Strauss AL (1967) *The Discovery of Grounded Theory: Strategies for Qualitative Research.* New York: Aldine.

Goldsmith M (1996) *Hearing the Voice of People with Dementia: Opportunities and Obstacles.* London: Jessica Kingsley Publishers.

Gubrium JF (1987) Structuring and destructuring the course of illness: the Alzheimer's disease experience. *Sociology of Health and Illness* 9(1), 1-24.

Harvath TA (1994) Interpretation and management of dementia-related behaviour problems. *Clinical Nursing Research* 3(1), 7-26.

Keady J and Nolan MR (1994) Younger-onset dementia: developing a longitudinal model as the basis for a research agenda and as a guide to interventions with sufferers and carers. *Journal of Advanced Nursing* 19, 659-669.

Keady J and Nolan MR (1995a) IMMEL1: assessing coping responses in the early stages of dementia. *British Journal of Nursing* 4(6), 309-314.

Keady J and Nolan MR (1995b) IMMEL 2: working to augment coping responses in early stages dementia. *British Journal of Nursing* 4(7), 377-380.

Keady J and Nolan MR (1995c) A stitch in time: facilitating proactive interventions with dementia caregivers: the role of community practitioners. *Journal of Psychiatric and Mental Health Nursing* 2(1), 33-40.

Keady J and Nolan MR (1996) Behavioural and instrumental stressers in dementia (BISID): refocussing the assessment of caregiver need in dementia. *Journal of Psychiatric and Mental Health Nursing* 3(3), 163-172.

LeNavenec C (1995) Understanding the Social Context of Families Experiencing Dementia: A Qualitative Approach. Paper presented at the 3rd European Conference of Gerontology, September, Amsterdam.

Sabat SR and Harré R (1992) The construction and deconstruction of self in Alzheimer's Disease. *Ageing and Society* 12(4), 443-461.

Taraborrelli P (1993) Exemplar A: becoming a carer. In Gilbert N (ed) *Researching Social Life.* London: Sage, 172-186.

Wilson HS (1989a) Family caregivers: the experience of Alzheimer's disease. *Applied Nursing Research* 2(1), 40-45.

Wilson HS (1989b) Family caregiving for a relative with Alzheimer's dementia: coping with negative choices. *Nursing Research* 38(2), 94-98.

Wuest J, Ericson PK and Stern PN (1994) Becoming strangers: the changing family caregiving relationship in Alzheimer's disease. *Journal of Advanced Nursing* 20, 437-443.

Yale R (1996) *Developing Support Groups for Individuals with Early-Stage Alzheimer's Disease: Planning, Implementation and Evaluation.* London: Jessica Kingsley.

7 Confidences: the experience of writing with people with dementia

John Killick

I start from a position of confidence. I am confident that it is possible to communicate with a person with dementia. I am confident that I will be able to write down what they have to say. I am confident that what they have to say will be coherent and illuminating.

So I am taking a number of leaps into the dark. But I am confident because so often my confidence has been rewarded. In my work as a writer in residence with people with dementia I now have hundreds of transcripts of meaningful conversations.

I do not set the agenda. I go with the person and their concerns (often literally as well, moving as they move). And so I can also be reasonably confident that what insights emerge have not been coerced out of them, or are reflections of my own concerns.

The unedited transcripts are of interest in themselves. They mirror the movement of people's minds. They often reveal worries or practical problems which can be addressed. But I don't always leave the texts in a raw state. Where I can perceive a thread of narrative or of feeling surrounded by other matter which does not seem relevant to the core issue I attempt to pare away what I judge to be inessential, leaving the primary material standing clear. This is what any editor does, of course, or a writer working with the product of his own creative processes, but in this unique circumstance I have to exercise extreme sensitivity both to language and idea. I have a rule-of-thumb principle never to add anything to the original, only to take away. The resulting piece of writing often emerges in the form of a poem.

This is not the place in which to speculate on why this might be so. Only to state that as a poet myself I recognise so often in this material the essential qualities of the art: assonance, alliteration, rhyme, rhythm, cadence and metaphor. Such poems can sometimes stand proudly beside those of professional writers. I shall give three examples.

The speaker of 'Sad Refrains' is Scottish, as the language patterns instantly proclaim; she is also despairing. Her confusion and grief find expression in statements which are balanced against each other. The statements are often completed within the line. There is a formality about her utterances which may be Biblical in origin, as she is obviously religious; it certainly acts as a stay against the anxiety she feels. But above all there are repetitions, often of phrases sometimes of sentences. These impart an inexorable quality to the text, and help to convince the reader of the force of emotion behind the words:

Sad Refrains

I've greet 'n greet 'n greet 'n greet...
was aye one for singing in the Chapel.
We were a' guid singers in ma family.
'There is a green hill far awa'.
I've aye been in a Christian place a' ma life.

I hope it a' comes quicker'n I think.

I dinna ken whit I've done. I dinna ken
whit I'm daein' sittin' here. I'm shair
ma man's in the hoose. And ma daughters.
And their bairns. I aye like wee ones to carry to.

I've greet 'n greet 'n greet 'n greet...

I wouldna be beholden to naebody.
I wouldna interfere wi' naebody's business.
I wouldna hurt naebody, no' me.
So why'm I nae hame? I've been here nearly a' day.

I hope it a' comes quicker'n I think.

We've a' been set up as Christian pedants
And ma mither wi' ainly one leg.
I wouldna hurt a hair. I wouldna hurt a bairn.
I've aye been in a Christian place a' ma life.

I've greet 'n greet 'n greet 'n greet...

It's gettin' dark. I've been here nearly a' day.
I havena a purse nor naethin'. I dinna ken
whit I've done. I've done naethin'.
I'll hae to be gettin' back to ma man.

I hope it a' comes quicker'n I think.

Note: to greet is to cry .

The speaker of the next poem is less put upon by circumstances. She retains a forthrightness, even tartness, of utterance. She has not lost a sense of her own identity, or her own empowerment – actually she rejoices in throwing that self-confidence playfully in the face of the writer. She is determined to hang on to what is essential in her own experience: It is mine. It is mine. And yet in doing so she reveals much of her own character which the dementia may have attacked but has been unable to break down. She too balances statements against each other, but mockingly, almost triumphantly. Whenever I read these lines I can hear that quality in her voice as she uttered them:

Battle of Wills

I don't mind you writing it down...
I can always alter it.

Of course I like there to be noise...
I wouldn't like to be talking to you
with nothing on the top!
Who are you? A gentleman?
No, go and look for one

I lived on a farm. I still do.
It is higher up than this.
I'd take you there
but I wouldn't want to take you there
to start with. It is mine. It is mine

There's nothing to say about the farm.
It's never still. Sometimes I live there,
and sometimes I don't.
Either on the farm,
or not on the farm.
I live there on my own
if there's no-one there with me.

Have you seen Jackie's dog?
What kind? You'd know what kinds
it wasn't if you saw it!

Can you swim without water?
I do, every time just before I go to bed.

Between you and me, you know,
it's a battle of wills.
Why don't you just lose first

Well, you'd better go home.
Wherever that is.
For the time being.

The speaker of the third poem cannot complete her sentences. She is at a later stage of competence in her use of language than those of the previous two poems. She is a person continually on the move, hence her references to 'I'm just off' or 'I'll just see'. There are mysterious phrases like 'up and down the language' and images (the one about the young girls wearing white). Nevertheless this gives a patterning to the writing which creates a poetic effect. But the piece contains two of the most affecting lines of any that have been given to me by those with whom I have worked. The sixth verse is profoundly moving however you interpret it: whether you think it is the other side of language, or the other side of mental coherence, that she is referring to, or (as is often the case with poetry) both at once:

On The Other Side

I'm just going to see what's round the corner...

I've lived here twenty-five weeks in the city,
up and down the language, twice up and down...
I'd better just have another look...

I'll tell you if you can understand the language.
And I'm talking, talking, talking all the time...

I'm just off to see if it's changed at all...

I didn't know if you would understand,
with you living on the other side...

I'll just see if it's all right over there...

Young girls wearing white on the other side
of their dress, getting married...

I'll just see if I can get far enough along...

Working as a writer with people with dementia is a humbling experience. To see the struggle for expression on people's faces, to hear the sounds tumbling over themselves in an effort to become words, phrases, sentences – this is painful. But when communication has been achieved, when the individual has leaped across the barrier to attain an utterance which embodies an insight – this is inspiriting, often for both parties. At such moments I am aware of the privilege that has been vouchsafed to me. I am aware too of another meaning of the word 'confidence' – that of a shared intimacy. And I remember the precept of another person with whom I worked on a number of occasions: 'Anything you can tell people about how things are for me is important'. It is in that spirit that I offer these writings.

Further reading

Killick J (1994) *Please Give Me Back My Personality!* Stirling: Dementia Services Development Centre.

8 The uniqueness of persons in dementia

Tom Kitwood

If I were to choose one issue that marks out good care from bad, the new culture from the old, it would be that of appreciating the uniqueness of persons. I would want all staff to do this for each man and woman in their care, and to commit themselves to it with both knowledge and feeling.

> *A manager is showing a possible new care assistant round the home. 'We've got five dementias in this home. Three of them cause very little trouble, especially the one that is bedfast. This one, though, can be very aggressive, and she sometimes attacks the other residents. This one is a smearer, I'm not sure whether we'll be able to keep her here much longer.' So saying, the manager points to two women who are asleep, slumped in their chairs. Both have recently received their morning dose of sedative medication.*

Why has there been such a devastating eradication of personhood? Why has there been such a marked discrimination? It would be comforting if we could say that an episode like this is a thing of the past, part of a culture of care that has had its day. Unfortunately this is not the case.

The truth is that while the leading edge of dementia care has made huge advances in recent years, the greater mass still lags far behind. The 'old culture' is still very much in place, but dispersed more widely than before, now that many of the older institutions of geriatric confinement have been closed. Much lipservice is paid to designing care in a way that respects the uniqueness of persons; but if we look at the reality rather than the propaganda, far less has changed than we might have hoped.

If the uniqueness of persons is to be fully appreciated, two things are necessary; neither is sufficient on its own.

Personal knowledge

It is now over ten years since several pioneers first highlighted the importance of life history for care practice. They showed that when the details of a person's past are known, many new possibilities for engagement are opened up, based on a true knowledge of that person's interests, tastes and experience; also, many enigmatic or difficult aspects of behaviour acquire a meaning. Far too little attention is being given to this matter; and even when some attempt has been made, the detail that would really help is often missing.

Here is a small example. A colleague and I were in a day centre, doing Dementia Care Mapping. One of the clients was acting strangely, almost as if he was trying to do some form of 'work'. I asked the manager what his job had been. She didn't know, but went to consult the records, and came back with the information that he had worked for 'Bowaters'. Neither she, her staff, nor I were any the wiser. Had he been a papermaking operative, a warehouseman, an HGV driver, one of the security staff, or what? His body movements remained without interpretation, and so never became actions in the full sense.

So, let us return to the two women with whom we began. How different the whole scenario might have been if staff had known the following facts. The first woman, Joan, had a long career as a teacher and had been deputy head of a junior school; her husband had been an engineer. Their marriage had been largely a formality, with frequent periods of separation while he was 'away on business', travelling abroad. Their son, after a promising beginning, had become involved in drugs. His marriage had collapsed, after which he became a very heavy drinker and went seriously 'off the rails'. Their daughter had then distanced herself from the family, leaving Joan very much alone. Much of Joan's later life had been marked by disappointments of this kind. If even these bare facts had been known, Joan's aggressive outbursts would have had a context, and there might have been a more serious attempt to meet her need.

Suppose the staff had known the following about the second woman, Annie. Her mother had died when she was aged 16. Her marriage lasted for only five years, from 1933 to 1938, when her husband, her son aged 3 and her daughter aged 2 were all killed in an accident. She had always lived near the poverty line, and her only occupation had been that of a cleaner. Around 1960 a new man came into her rather lonely life, but he died about two years after she met him. Not long after that there was another man; he dominated her, 'made use of her' and there were suspicions of sexual abuse. With knowledge of this kind it would be almost impossible to label Annie as a 'smearer'. She would be seen as a real human being who had lived through dreadful privation, and who deserved comfort and compassion in her final years.

Empathy

This, then, is the second essential for appreciating the uniqueness of persons. Empathy means having an understanding of both of what another is experiencing, and of their manner of experiencing. Empathy is not primarily a matter of intellect; it is a form of understanding that centres on feeling and intuition. For most people, developing empathic skill requires a profound inner change; growing into a much greater degree of inner peace and self-acceptance than is common in our culture. Also an empathic relationship doesn't just happen; it requires time, commitment and communication.

Eric is a tall, well-built, distinguished looking man. He might be taken as a senior doctor, or a managing director. He is courteous and agreeable in his manner. Anyone who draws close to him with empathy would soon sense that he is using great effort to ward off a deep sense of personal catastrophe. He is exceedingly vulnerable, hypersensitive, desperately afraid of losing control; yet he does not want to upset other people, or to impose his troubles on anyone else. What will happen if people around him assume from his appearance that all is well? What if the sense of catastrophe overwhelms him? Only if someone gains a sense of what he is really experiencing will it be possible to help him through his existential crisis.

Irene is a tiny woman, rather tense in body, her face is haggard, and she hardly ever smiles. She spends a lot of time walking around, on her own, apparently living in her own private world. Anyone who takes the trouble to be truly available to her will get a huge surprise. They will find someone who is extremely warm-hearted, waiting to give of herself. The grasp of her hand is firm; her body, though small, is strong. She is a person of great courage, and she is dealing with her disabilities as best she can. We get the sense that she is a fighter; perhaps she has often had to fight, for her own survival and that of those whom she loves. She causes no trouble, so she is often forgotten; but she is fighting still. If she were truly noticed, she would soon flourish, and the warmth and richness of her personality might bring great happiness to others.

Maintaining personhood

In the worst kind of care settings – those that epitomise the old culture of care – thousands of men and women were denied the privilege of personhood. They became little more than a cardboard cut-out: an instance of some psychiatric category, or a particular kind of nuisance to care staff. The vegetative state in which so many of them ended their lives can hardly be attributed to a simple neurological process.

If personhood is to be maintained, it is essential that each individual be appreciated in his or her uniqueness. Where there is empathy without personal knowledge, care will be aimless and unfocused. Where there is personal knowledge without empathy, care will be detached and cold. But when empathy and personal knowledge are brought together, miracles can happen.

Note

The biographical material here is based on my own life history work, but for the sake of confidentiality all names are fictitious and some minor details have been changed.

9 Why should family caregivers feel guilty?

Robert T Woods

Caregivers are saints?

It is widely recognised that families of people with dementia provide the bulk of dementia care in the United Kingdom and in most other countries. It is clear that if family care were to be removed, the community support services made available through the statutory authorities would collapse. However, it is also well established that caring at home for somebody suffering from a dementing condition can be a very difficult task (see for example Zarit and Edwards, 1996). As well as the day-to-day difficulties of providing care for someone who may need a great deal of supervision and help with physical tasks such as dressing, feeding and toileting, there is also the emotional strain of seeing the often devastating change in someone with whom the carer has had a relationship for many years. In dementia especially, the care recipient may not acknowledge their need for care and so may at times be an unwilling participant in daily care tasks. For some caregivers there may be a number of difficult and demanding aspects of the person's behaviour with which to cope, such as verbal or physical aggression, wandering, shouting and repeated questions.

In carrying out research or clinical work with such family caregivers over the years, I personally have never failed to be impressed by the commitment, dedication, resilience and coping resources which are brought to this difficult task. Such sentiments are widely shared. For example, in their extensive longitudinal study of the caregiving careers of family members looking after somebody suffering from a dementia, Aneshensel et al (1995) write:

> at a historical time and in a society in which people are presumably driven by motives of self-gratification, care-givers as a group outstandingly embody many of the best humanitarian values... For many people, then, care-giving is an expression of extreme altruism, where one's own well-being is sacrificed for the benefit of another.

There is a tendency amongst researchers and professionals, and in society as a whole, to canonise family caregivers, recognising the enormous contribution which they make to society, at some cost to themselves and often in quite difficult circumstances. In a just society then, family caregivers would feel pride regarding their contribution and their role.

In fact, far from feeling esteem and satisfaction many family caregivers experience a strong sense of strain and burden. An aspect of this which has been largely unreflected in the caregiving research literature, but which will create lively discussion at any carers' group, is that of guilt. Guilt may be thought of as the emotional state produced by internal recognition of a violation of internalised moral standards, a self-administered punishment. While not all family caregivers experience guilt, there are indications that a substantial proportion of caregivers at some point do experience this emotion in relation to their caregiving. For example, Nolan and Grant (1992) reported that over half of their sample of carers had problems with guilt. Clearly a great many carers do not see themselves as saints.

There is another side to family care, which although highly relevant is often considered as a separate topic from family caregiving. There is increasing awareness of elder abuse, which includes instances of people with dementia being maltreated by members of their family. This mistreatment may be physical, sexual, psychological, or financial and may include acts of commission (abuse) or omission (neglect) (Kingston and Reay, 1996).

It is important to reflect that the family caregiving scenario can be one where the highest human values are manifested or one where degradation may hold sway. Yet it would be stretching the definitions of elder abuse beyond any sensible limits to equate caregivers' feelings of guilt from having let the person with dementia down in some way with the abusive situation. Caregivers are ordinary human beings and guilt is an everyday emotion in the world of human relationships.

Institutional placement

Guilt has often been particularly highlighted in relation to the decision to place the person with dementia in some form of institutional care. For example, Aneshensel et al (1995) reported an increase in guilt feelings among family carers where the person with dementia had been admitted to institutional care.

Nolan and Grant (1992) indicate that even where the person is placed only temporarily in institutional care, as in a respite admission, guilt feelings may be prevalent. They describe three factors which appear to influence guilt in their sample of carers. These were:

- the reaction of the elderly person themselves to the respite admission;
- the perceived inadequacy of the institution providing the respite care;
- the perception that staff failed to recognise the carer's expert knowledge of the elderly person.

The quality of the institution may influence each of these factors, and there is some evidence that higher quality may be associated with a lower level of guilt among family caregivers. For example, in Australia, Wells and Jorm (1987) reported no increase in guilt feelings when the person was admitted to a high quality special care unit for people with dementia. Woods and Macmillan (1994) showed a reduction in guilt following the move of the elderly person with dementia from a distant Victorian asylum to a purpose-built, local, homely unit. However, the association in this study between guilt and distress arising from the changes in the person with dementia, and the importance of the elderly person's reaction to respite care noted above, suggest factors other than the institutional environment are having an impact. One relative remarked how it was only after her husband had been in the special care unit for three or four months that she began to notice how pleasant it was; previously her attention had been so preoccupied with the immense change in her husband's function and abilities. It is important to endeavour to improve the quality of institutions, and this may have some effect on caregivers' guilt, but the changes in the relationship between caregiver and person with dementia brought about by the onset and progress of the disease may continue to be a major influence.

Guilt in relationships

If guilt is not simply a result of the decision to institutionalise the person with dementia, guilt feelings should be evident among relatives of people with dementia being cared for at home. The focus of these guilt feelings may be slightly different, perhaps relating more to the evident difficulty of meeting all the person's needs single-handed in the home situation, rather than to a sense of letting the person down, arising from the decision to allow the person to enter an institution. Although the literature is relatively sparse on this topic, it does appear that, in common with feelings of strain, guilt may well be present both before and after institutionalisation. It certainly does not arise anew after the person enters institutional care. Caregiving is a complex, demanding task, and, as in so much of human relating, it is always possible to reflect on how one might have done things differently and on mistakes that have been made. Indeed some carers blame themselves even for aspects of the person's disease, or perhaps feel guilt that they did not recognise it earlier, or that they saw it merely as an extension of the person's previous style of behaviour.

Guilt arises in the context of what may be a long standing relationship, perhaps that of marriage or of parent-child. The extent to which the caregiver experiences guilt will depend both on their own natural propensity for self-blame and the particular relationship dynamic, which may have such a lengthy history as to operate at an automatic level, without the caregiver being consciously aware of the process.

These considerations indicate that there is a need to develop more refined ways of considering the experience of guilt and of the relationship pattern in caregiving research. Measurements in this area have tended to be unsophisticated. For example, Aneshensel et al used a five item guilt scale comprising two items relating to the relationship with the person before the onset of the condition, two relating to letting the person down currently and the fifth item being a global rating of guilt. Woods and Macmillan (1994) used visual analogue scales of guilt frequency and severity. Others have used perhaps a single item to assess guilt or a measure of propensity to guilt rather than guilt related to caregiving per se.

A more detailed examination is required to indicate the extent guilt feelings do change in their focus after placement.

The framework proposed by Motenko (1989) for the reasons and meaning underlying caregiving would also benefit from examination in relation to guilt feelings. Three primary motives were put forward:

- reciprocity – the caregiver is motivated by a debt of gratitude for affection and care received previously;

- a sense of duty, obligation or responsibility;
- tender loving care – the caregiver feels able to offer the best care for the person.

Where the caregiver provides care purely out of a sense of duty, one might expect guilt feelings to be most evident. Certainly it is here that a sense of 'role captivity', described by Aneshensel et al (1985) as being the main predictor of placement, is likely to be most apparent. However, it would be perhaps mistaken to view reasons for caregiving as only arising from the past relationship. Current mutuality and satisfaction from the caregiving role itself must also be considered. One of the important ways in which the caregiving research literature is currently developing is to give more recognition to the satisfaction many do receive from caregiving, with strain, distress and burden by no means reflecting the totality of the experience.

Gilbert et al (1994) have described how, from an evolutionary perspective, guilt may be seen as having evolved as a self-monitoring system to motivate help-giving, to avoid harm to, or exploitation of, others. Guilt involves letting others down in some way and motivates reparations. In this framework guilt is seen as the driving force of all caregiving. Not all caregivers experience it; many have found ways of satisfying their internal standards and expectations. This may be through a sense of reciprocity in the relationship, that their care is appreciated and has purpose, or through a sense that they are able to provide care better than anyone else; this may motivate the reluctance on the part of many to consider institutional care. Those who set themselves higher standards are most likely to perceive themselves as having failed to live up to their own expectations. Indeed these very expectations may have been established in the context of the relationship with the care-recipient, and fall into a life-long pattern of letting the person down, never quite living up to the standards expected.

Caregivers feel guilt for many reasons. It is not simply that the caregiver has placed or is considering placing the person in an institution or respite care; nor is it just that the caregiver has at times lost their temper or not matched society's saintly stereotype; nor that they have taken upon themselves the burden of responsibility for the onset and progress of the dementing condition. All these are important factors, but it is suggested that of overriding significance is the difficulty in finding ways of attenuating within a particular long-standing relationship the feelings of guilt which have evolved precisely to motivate helping the other. Perhaps most remarkable is the way in which so many carers are able to find meaning and satisfaction within a relationship and so reduce to a manageable level these potentially pervasive and distressing feelings.

References

Aneshensel CS, Pearlin LI, Mullan JT, Zarit SH and Whitlatch CJ (1995) *Profiles in Caregiving: the Unexpected Career.* San Diego: Academic Press.

Gilbert P, Pehl J and Allan S (1994) The phenomenology of shame and guilt: an empirical investigation. *British Journal of Medical Psychology* 67, 23-36.

Kingston P and Reay A (1996). Elder abuse and neglect. In Woods RT (ed) *Handbook of the Clinical Psychology of Ageing.* Chichester: Wiley, 423-438.

Motenko AK (1989) The frustrations, gratifications and well-being of dementia care-givers. *Gerontologist* 29, 166-172.

Nolan M and Grant G (1992) *Regular Respite.* London: Age Concern England.

Wells Y and Jorm AF (1987) Evaluation of a special nursing home unit for dementia sufferers: a randomised controlled comparison with community care. *Australian and New Zealand Journal of Psychiatry* 21, 524-531.

Woods RT and Macmillan M (1994) Home at last? Impact of a local 'homely' unit for dementia sufferers on their relatives. In Challis D, Davies B and Traske K (eds) *Community Care: New Agendas and Challenges from the UK and Overseas.* Aldershot: Ashgate, 75-85.

Zarit SH and Edwards AB (1996) Family caregiving: research and clinical intervention. In Woods RT (ed) *Handbook of the Clinical Psychology of Ageing.* Chichester: Wiley, 333-368.

Policies and services

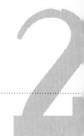

10 Social Services Inspectorate inspection of services for older people with dementia in the community

Derek Brown

The Department of Health's Social Services Inspectorate conducted an inspection of services for older people with dementia in the community in eight local authorities in England between September 1995 and March 1996.

We looked at social care agencies' capacities to respond appropriately to older people with dementia who live alone in the community or with carers. We sought to evaluate the ways in which older people with dementia are enabled, according to their abilities, to participate and exercise choices in the community care assessment and care management processes. We also examined the quality of services delivered to maintain service users in the community and the extent to which these supported carers. This included services provided by the independent sector.

The quality of arrangements between personal social service and health providers are crucial to the support of this client group. Because of this, we paid attention to the multidisciplinary working arrangements for diagnosis, assessment and collaboration in delivering care plans.

Fieldwork was underpinned by a survey of fifty active cases in each authority and analysis of this material will inform our report. Our methodology included interviews with social services departments, health and independent services managers and practitioners, carers, and visits to sites providing services. Each inspection team was assisted in its work by a senior nurse from a NHS regional office or health trust and by a Lay Assessor.

We found that best practice appears to occur where there are good collaborative arrangements between staff from the social services department, the NHS and the independent sector who are content to blur the boundaries of their activities, whether or not this is supported by competent strategies and planning arrangements. Most people with dementia were dependent on what generic services for older people could provide, and inspectors found few specialist services, although where these did exist they were generally of high quality.

A report of the inspection will be available in 1997.

Further information

Available from the author of the report: Derek Brown, Inspector, Social Service Inspectorate, Tyne Bridge Tower, Church Street, Gateshead NE8 2DU.

11 EACH: European Alzheimer Clearing House

Leen Meulenbergs

The aims

The European Alzheimer Clearing House (EACH) aims at making better use of existing information and expertise (clearing) and putting forward 'examples of good practice' in the field of care for patients with Alzheimer's Disease and Related Disorders (ADRD).

Rather than undertaking the ambitious and probably impossible task of covering the entire field, EACH will focus on a limited number of priority projects of high importance for patients and carers, specially in ADRD care but also in public health in general, and thus effecting a significant impact on the field.

Priority projects

- training;
- good practices;
- Alzheimer associations;
- socioeconomic impact;
- ethical issues;
- support programs;
- nursing qualifications;
- substance counselling;
- clinical aspects.

Overall, EACH is willing to contribute substantially in the field of information, education and policy development in as much as they relate to the

European Union Public Health Policy in favour of persons suffering from ADRD.

An integrated approach

In general, the programme and the tasks consist of:
- defining the priorities;
- active outreach to get all relevant information in the EU member states;
- analysis and restructuring of information in collaboration with national experts and international networks;
- producing results, well targeted on the specific end users such as patients, families, professional caregivers, trainers, volunteers, policy makers at different levels, mass media and others;
- user friendly and economic dissemination of the results such as workbooks, training manuals, brochures, appropriate use of 'new media' such as Internet, ao;
- evaluation of the efficiency and effectiveness of the project, including a reassessment of priorities.

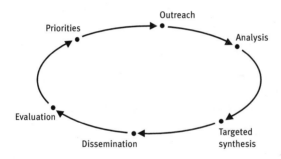

A developing project within a community framework

An end product of the EACH project is much more than the sum of its components. Instead of conducting fragmented tasks within different sectors, disciplines and society levels, EACH focuses on an integrated approach likely to decrease costs and increase efficiency and, consequently, benefits for the ADRD care receivers and caregivers.

A goal-oriented collaboration with the task leaders, and participants is organised in order to assure strong interaction (interdisciplinary, intersectorial, cross-cultural) and to benefit optimally from each others work and experience.

The end products will contribute to: a more integrated (non fragmented) approach, increased public awareness, improved services, higher quality of life for patients and their families, empowerment of self help, policy development and, fundamentally, a proper balance between member state specifics and a European common core.

The mission of EACH

The mission of EACH is to collect, analyse, compile, disseminate and promote application of:

- knowledge of Alzheimer's Disease and Related Disorders, and their consequences;
- optimal ways of management for such patients, their families, caregivers, administrators, decision makers and the general public;
- knowledge-based care to achieve the highest possible level of living and quality of life for patients and their families.

Further information

European Alzheimer Clearing House, Esplanade Building, 3rd floor – room 303, Avenue Pachéco 19, B-1010 Brussels, Belgium. Telephone: (+32) 2 210 44 62, Fax: (+32) 2 218 67 46, e-mail: each@health.fgov.be, http://www.each.be.

12 Taking dementia services in Victoria into the twenty-first century

Rosemary Calder

What do we want for people with dementia and their carers?

- recognition of the abilities, preferences, and contributions of people with dementia and their carers;
- an environment in which the rights and needs of people with dementia and their carers are recognised and met;
- universal community acceptance and understanding of dementia and the dementing process;
- universal recognition of and response to the needs of people with dementia from all health and community services providers;

- ready availability and access to comprehensive clinical assessment and diagnosis for people with dementia and their carers;
- services which enable carers to obtain and manage the support they need including access to appropriate education and training;
- access to appropriate support services and continuity of care throughout the pathway of the dementing process; and
- individualised care management in programs which are responsive and flexible over time.

What needs to change?

- the lack of universal recognition of people with dementia as equal members of the community;
- the lack of recognition and of respect for the dignity of people with dementia, their carers and their individual needs;
- the dearth of information given to people with dementia and their carers, relatives and supporters;
- the lack of service provider understanding of the dementing process and its impact on people and carers over time, and their limited contractual commitment to providing support and services appropriate to the changing needs of dementing people and carers;
- the capacity of the service system to respond quickly and effectively to expressed needs and circumstances of people with dementia and their carers;
- the inequitable distribution of dementia services within Victoria; and
- the lack of development of care plans including provision of counselling services for both people with dementia and caregivers.

What do we want for, from and of professional and non-professional providers?

- recognition that dementia is a major public health issue and the responsibility of every segment of the health and community service system;
- commitment to ongoing professional education, skills development and monitoring;
- recognition of the responsibilities of professional providers in supporting both the current and future needs of the carer; and
- commitment to continuity of care for the person with dementia.

The Ministerial Task Force for Dementia Services in the State of Victoria in Australia proposed these answers to the following questions: 'What do we want for people with dementia and their carers? What needs to change?' and 'What do we want for, from, and of professional providers and carers?' The task force was established in November 1995 to thoroughly review the services provided to people with dementia and their carers, establish standards for best practice for service providers and identify their educational and training needs.

Victoria is a small, highly urbanised southern state of Australia. Its population is projected to grow from 4.5 million people in 1996 to 4.9 million people in 2011.[1]

The Victorian population is ageing, with those aged 70 years and over expected to increase from 157,600 people in 1996 to 203,600 people in the year 2011.[2]

Thirty-one per cent of Victorians live in rural areas and 69 per cent live in metropolitan areas. Along with the rise in the absolute numbers of people aged 70 years and over, there will be an increase in the number of people with dementia in Victoria. While the prevalence rate will not change, absolute numbers of people with dementia will increase over the next fifteen years. The total estimated prevalence for dementia for those aged 70 years and over will rise from about 31,000 people in 1996 to about 44,000 people in 2011.[3]

Overview of policy development for dementia services in Australia

The work of the Ministerial Task Force on Dementia Services in Victoria built on and expanded the work started by the National Action Plan for Dementia Care (NAPDC), launched in August 1992 by the then Australian Commonwealth Department of Health, Housing and Community Services (DHHCS). The NAPDC provided funding and a five year strategic framework (from 1992/93 to 1996/97) aimed at strengthening the existing Australia-wide service response to people with dementia and their carers and to identify service gaps. As the Commonwealth government had primary responsibility for the funding and provision of nursing home services and the major responsibility for the broader range of aged care services through the National Home and Community Care Program (HACC), it was essential that this initial reform be driven by the Commonwealth with cooperation from the States.

The NAPDC grew out of recommendations made in the 1990-91 Commonwealth Mid-Term Review of the Aged Care Reform Strategy. The Aged Care Reform Strategy provided the initial impetus for the explicit recognition of the particular needs of people with dementia and their carers in the health and community service system through the HACC program, and through reform of the operation and funding of nursing homes and hostels. The mid-term review also recognised the need for a more coordinated service response to people with dementia rather than the continuing development of ad hoc services.

The Victorian aged care system had also undergone rapid reform and realignment over the four years from 1992 to 1996. The State Government reduced investment in inadequate and inappropriate residential care services and significantly increased specialist geriatric health services, particularly rehabilitation, and in-home care and support. These State based reforms, and the conclusion of the NAPDC, provided the basis for the examination of future dementia care issues and needs by the Dementia Task Force.

In this context, the State Minister for Aged Care and the Department of Human Services wished to take a more strategic approach to the provision of dementia services across the service system.

The task force

The Minister for Aged Care, Robert Knowles, established the Ministerial Task Force on Dementia Services in Victoria in December 1995. Its role was to advise on the best ways to further develop and coordinate effective dementia care and support services in the State. The task force drew on the expertise of individuals with a significant background and knowledge of the issues and practices associated with dementia care. It was established specifically to review the range of services needed by people with dementia and their carers in the community and across areas such as assessment, acute hospitals, psychogeriatric services and residential care settings. Coordination of services across the entire health system was required. Members formed three working parties to address the three areas outlined in the task force terms of reference which were:

- to advise on strategies for the development of integrated dementia services for Victoria which encompass acute, outpatient, community and home based programs;
- to advise on a set of suitable performance and outcome measures for monitoring agency performance;
- to advise on strategies to ensure workforce development, education and training at both agency and postgraduate level.

The target group

Although dementia may result from more than seventy medical and surgical conditions, the task force focused primarily on those dementias that occur within the older population such as Alzheimer's type, vascular dementias, idiopathic and miscellaneous dementias including Pick's and Jakob-Creutzfeldt syndrome.

The task force recognised that it was essential to view the needs of the carer and the client concurrently throughout the course of the disease recognising the different, but specific, health needs of the carer. Carers were defined as including unpaid family members, friends or neighbours who provided care and assistance for a person with dementia. They were distinguished from professional, 'paid' or volunteer caregivers who provide care and support in a formal capacity, usually through a service agency.

Pathway of dementia

Continuity of care was identified as an important but often missing component of care for people with dementia and their carers. The task force recognised that the person with dementia living in the community was likely to make use of a range of different services. These could include consultations with general practitioners, diagnostic services, episodic acute care, pharmaceutical services; community care services such as district nursing, home help and respite care; adult day care, residential care, financial services, transport and income security. Service needs could vary over the course of the disease. The task force's approach was to focus on how the person with dementia and the carer interacted with the service system, and to identify the critical points over the long-term pathway followed by the progress of the disease at which problems for people with dementia and their carers can occur. The task force identified five points along the pathway at which integration of services became critical. The service integration working party looked at the services, key issues and problems relevant at each of these points:

- early identification;
- contact with and need for acute services;
- access to non-dementia specific services for person with dementia and their carer;
- formal care and support system introduced;
- decision to transfer to residential care.

The task force was particularly interested in those parts of the service system that were the responsibility of the State Government and were problematic for consumers.

There had been some attempt in the past in Victoria to incorporate dementia-specific outcomes into existing service standards but there were no generally accepted sets of performance indicators focused exclusively on the needs of people with dementia and their carers. The task force aimed to raise awareness about best practice across the service system, not just among service providers who frequently cared for people with dementia or who had developed standards. A quality assurance approach which encouraged self monitoring by service providers was considered the most promising. Through a process of consultation the working party on performance indicators developed generic sets of standards and performance indicators for widespread circulation to service providers. The task force will promote these 'ideal' standards and indicators for adoption and further development by individual agencies to suit their own particular clientele and circumstances.

Closely allied to the process of quality assurance is the need to increase knowledge, change attitudes and develop skills of service providers so that they can respond effectively to the needs of people with dementia and their carers. The development, education and training working party identified the knowledge and skill gaps and attitudinal changes required of all service providers who come into contact with people with dementia and their carers in all parts of the Victorian service system. Gaps were identified in existing educational and training programs offered and their effectiveness in preparing service providers for their caring role were evaluated. The working party proposed ways in which existing courses and programs could be strengthened and developed new strategies to target identified gaps. Appropriate implementation strategies for different groups of service providers ranging from general practitioners to the service provider dealing with the person over the bank counter were proposed.

Task force outcomes

The task force produced a number of discussion papers on dementia care issues including background, service integration, performance indicators, education and training, community awareness, carers strategy and public health strategy papers. They outlined strategies for dissemination and consultation through the health and community support system, professional organisations, academic bodies, the general community and consumer and advocacy sector.

The task force's final report to the Minister in February 1997 entitled 'Identifying the Issues: the way forward' outlines the key outcomes of the work of the task force based on the previous papers. The paper will provide the Minister with recommendations on standards of care, funding requirements and performance indicators, education and training requirements for implementation through the State Government's funding arrangements for aged care services.

Notes

1 Australian Bureau of Statistics Catalogue no 3222.0 Estimates based on ABS Projection Series A and B.

2 Australian Bureau of Statistics Catalogue no 3222.0 Estimates based on ABS Projection Series A.

3 Australian Bureau of Statistics Catalogue no 3222.0 Estimates based on ABS Projection Series A and B.

Further information

Aged Care Program, Department of Human Services, 10/555 Collins Street, Melbourne 3000, Victoria, Australia.

13 The art of the state: public policy in dementia care

Harry Cayton

The welfare state is undoubtedly old and frail. Some recommend major surgery. Some suggest merely keeping it warm and comfortable. For others euthanasia is the only rational option. But can the welfare state and particularly the health service be revived and rehabilitated? What part should the state have to play in dementia care as we move into the next century?

The truth is that for all their problems the health service, social care and social security systems have served the majority of people well. It is political rhetoric as much as real symptoms which has created a sense of crisis in the last few years; a sense of crisis which is more about the challenge to our social and economic values when faced with an ageing population than it is about the problems of the welfare state.

The political rhetoric has been backed by government action. The NHS and community care reforms have been primarily about controlling expenditure and reducing the scope of state involvement in health and social care. Health trusts have cut provision of health care for older people dramatically, particularly long term care for people with dementia, and social services are encouraged to provide only for those who would otherwise be admitted to resident or nursing homes. Both these developments have been encouraged by the government's steadfast refusal to establish national levels of provision or national eligibility criteria. In a recent speech Stephen Dorrell (1996), Secretary of State for Health looked forward to a time when social care would only be 'a safety net service' for those quite unable to provide for themselves and envisaged a growing role for family carers and 'voluntary activity' in providing community care. Health care is increasingly redefined as treatment and cure. Prevention, rehabilitation, and continuing care are no longer health but social care. The former is free at the point of delivery, the latter means-tested.

The consultation paper *A New Partnership for Care in Old Age* (1996) published by the government went further than before in proposing the development of a private insurance market, stimulated by government subsidy, to encourage individuals to insure against long term care costs.

The drive of current policy is clear: to reduce the role of the state, to reduce the tax cost, to shift responsibility to the individual or their family, to reduce nationally defined standards and regulations, to encourage local and independent sector provision.

In this financially rather than socially driven policy people with dementia and those who care for them seem particularly cruelly trapped by the convergence of reducing state provision and increasing need. The number of older people is growing (though it is not as the ageist slogans would have us believe a 'tidal wave', more a gentle swell) and in consequence the number of people with dementia is increasing too. There are however many more elements affecting the care needs of people with dementia in the next century than rising numbers.

Demographic patterns suggest much larger numbers of people living alone in old age. Smaller families, marriage breakdown, differences in life expectancy between men and women, geographical variation in the distribution of older people will all affect the kind of health and social care service we will need. There will be important developments in anti-dementia drugs in the next decade which may have a significant impact on an individual's ability to remain at home. The new more positive approach to dementia care will also have an effect on the balance of need between institutional and domestic care.

It seems ironic that just as professional and family caregivers, along with doctors and scientists are developing positive and constructive approaches to improving the quality of life of people with dementia, we have politicians and policy makers who seem to view older people as a burden on rather than an enrichment of our society.

The state acts on behalf of us all to promote both public and private good. Public policy should approach the issue of dementia care with positive aims. These should be concerned with quality, provision and access to care. The state is an effective vehicle for sharing cost, enabling access and availability, regulating and maintaining quality.

The all party Health Select Committee in its report on long term care (1996) states clearly, 'Funding long term care mainly from general taxation is a defensible option, which is both possible and affordable'. Indeed, as our health service has shown, it is possible to provide universal health care through taxation without spending a disproportionate amount because taxation shares the cost most effectively across the population as a whole. One only has to look to the private insurance model in the United States to see the problems both of inequality and cost which such a system creates. The NHS reforms of the early 1990s have already started to increase variation in quality and level of provision in the UK.

Universal provision needs to be matched by equality of access. The increasingly deregulated system of competing health trusts is producing wide variation in eligibility. National eligibility criteria for dementia care are needed and structural changes in the relationship between health and social care services must be made. The recent suggestion from the Royal College of Nursing that nursing care should be free at the point of delivery in whatever setting it is provided is worthy of serious consideration, as are proposals for the elimination of the distinction between residential and nursing homes and for the merging of the commissioning functions of health authorities and social service departments. The health and social care divide is one of the most destructive and unhelpful aspects of our present system made even more so by the internal market. It is absolutely a matter for the state to define and regulate such institutions and relationships.

Since the purpose of health and social care is improved quality of life for individuals and the community the state has a role in regulating and defining quality. To do so is to promote both private and public good: private good in that the individual's quality of life is enhanced, public good in improved health in the community and reduction on the overall burden of morbidity.

The widespread delivery of good practice in dementia care depends on the structure of our social institutions and the economic model of our society. The state has a vital role to play and fundamental responsibilities it cannot avoid. The art of the state should not be the avoidance of those responsibilities but the pursuit of the wellbeing of the individual and the community. For the next generation of older people there is no more important challenge for government than renewing the welfare state.

References

Dorrell S MP (1996) The challenge of social services, *Politeia* lecture, 8 July 1996.

HMSO (1996) *A New Partnership for Care in Old Age*. London: HMSO.

HMSO (1996) *Long-Term Care: Future Provision and Funding*. Health Committee Third Report, London: HMSO.

14 Pragmatic groups: interactions and relationships between people with dementia

Kate Foster

Introduction: therapeutic groups and pragmatic groups

This chapter argues that the social interactions between people with dementia, as well as with their caregivers, should be seen as an aspect of the quality of care. This is based on the assumption that social interactions are particularly important in influencing the wellbeing of people with dementia, both positively and negatively.

Specialist services bring people with dementia together in two kinds of groups. The first kind is 'therapeutic', where participants engage in a psychological therapy (see Bleathman and Morton, 1995). I am calling, for the purposes of this article, the second kind of group 'pragmatic'. This is where people are brought together to receive care, such as day care, medical assessment, respite for their informal carers, or residential care. Recipients meet in pragmatic groups because they share a need, which is professionally defined. Pragmatic groups give care collectively which is often cheaper and easier to organise than delivering it to individuals at home. Recipients are unlikely to be able to choose who else is in the group, but are likely to spend at least as much time with other clients as with staff. Generally in society independence, autonomy and individuality are prized. In pragmatic groups, the skills of communal living are needed, namely tolerance, sharing and sociability.

Given that there is no cure currently available, the main aims of caring for people with dementia are to provide as good a physical and social environment as possible. Practitioners and researchers are becoming more optimistic about what can be achieved by good quality care (see Kitwood and Bredin, 1992). Self-esteem can be improved by the right kind of social interaction, and this may help people to maintain their abilities better than they would otherwise (see Holden and Woods, 1995).

Social interaction can act both to promote and to diminish wellbeing. Jones (1991) suggests that to communicate successfully with people with dementia requires considerable skill and insight. Writing about 'learned helplessness',

Lubinski (1991 p142) made the premise that:

> *dementia is not only a real change in cognitive, emotional, and*
> *communicative behaviour but is also a learned behaviour*
> *emanating from the perceptions of those in the environment.*

Given the strengthening belief that patterns of social interaction can make both positive and negative differences to people with dementia, how successfully can people with dementia communicate with each other?

There has been little discussion of the consequences of gathering people with strangers who, like themselves, may have diminishing social skills as a result of their dementia. This article considers the way people with dementia get on with each other in pragmatic groups, and how such gatherings may also be 'therapeutic', and ideally, enjoyable. How older people get on together has been studied and used as a measure of social environment (Moos and Lemke, 1984); some attention has been paid to the way that staff interact with people with dementia (see Dean et al, 1993). Studies have looked at the way social and physical environments shape behaviour and interactions (see Netten, 1993), but little attention has been paid to the quality of relationships between people with dementia.

The ability of people with dementia to sustain relationships with their informal carers may be severely affected by their illness (Levin et al, 1989). We also learn that people with dementia can be unpopular in mixed settings, though this can depend on their personal characteristics (Wilkin and Hughes, 1987; Willcocks et al, 1987). This suggests that interactions and the development of relationships in pragmatic groups may be complicated by the process of dementia. Without discussion and research, we remain in a shadowy world of assumptions.

Case study of people with dementia in a pragmatic group: care housing

This section uses some of the findings (Foster, research in progress) of an evaluation of a form of group-living for people with dementia. The methods used included semi-structured interviews with twenty-eight staff members and observation.

Staff made some contradictory assumptions and observations. For example, on one hand staff said that: 'Dementia is a leveller'. On the other hand they thought that mixing people who have either more or less severe dementia could create problems. Staff believed that residents' social background – their class, wealth and ethnicity for example – did not really affect how they got on with each other. Against this, they said that residents could be very critical of each other. They were not sure if residents recognised each other, but knew that some had personality clashes and others had made friendships.

What appeared to be the case on closer examination? Interviews suggested that residents seemed more concerned with other people's behaviour that they found strange, than reassured by the fact that they all had dementia. Residents may have been afraid that they would become like the most severely affected people. One staff member described and commented on conversation between residents.

> For example, they will say: 'Oh look at her, pouring that into a sugar bowl!'; 'Oh for god's sake!'; They will sit and talk: 'Eating like a baby!'; 'Can you not use your fork right?'; 'You are silly, you should not be at table'; 'Shouldn't be here, should be in hospital'…
> They can be really rude, I think it's just a fear, and it is not nice, to watch someone who's mind can't coordinate itself, and who is possibly drooling – the others do have to witness it.

Residents did learn to recognise each other, though some had more difficulty than others, and generally perhaps it took longer than normal. A comment reportedly made by a resident about me when I was observing in the unit illustrates this point.

> That girl keeps coming in and out: the more I see her, the more I know her.

Residents could be helpful to each other. During observation in a unit, I watched two residents lay a table together, a task they did twice a day. They were friends, but Mrs Knox was more forgetful than Mrs Thomas.[1]

> Mrs Knox came from the kitchen with the cutlery and asked Mrs Thomas how many places to lay. Mrs Thomas said six, though actually four were needed, and they could not exactly work it out. They could not remember if they should lay the staff table or not. Mrs Thomas encouraged Mrs Knox to go ahead and lay her own place, and she put them down in a slightly odd way. Mrs Thomas asked Mrs Knox if she didn't think a desert spoon was rather big for her tea cup. Mrs Knox said that no, she thought it was OK. Mrs Thomas politely acquiesced. Later on in the meal, Mrs Knox was struggling with her desert spoon when she wanted to stir her tea. Mrs Thomas suggested that she used the other end of the spoon and this would do the job, which it did.

Friendships could form between the sexes as well, with residents having their preferred partners for dances and sing-songs. One woman used to tuck up a male resident in bed some times; staff said both enjoyed this.

If residents were critical of each other, this included everyday issues like who sat where, the way people spoke or dressed, or ate their food. Another reason why residents fell out was because their dementia made them misinterpret where they were, who the other people were, and what things belonged to them. The following vignettes come from interviews with staff who described how residents sometimes annoyed each other. The respondents own words are used insofar as possible.

- Residents can be quite rude sometimes to visitors. Mrs Seton for example, when we get one family in, who can be rough and talk slang, she can ask: 'Who is this trash?'
- Mr Edwards once accused Mr Wallace of having an affair with his wife and hit him. Mr Wallace said he didn't even know his wife. It was alarming for the care officer at the time…it was unexpected, during lunch.
- It can be difficult for people who lift things, like cups and handbags, or for people who are continually on the go, to fit in here. The other residents find it hard to accept, and try to constrain them to their seats.
- When one woman starts talking, other residents say: What are you talking about? When they can't follow what she says, they more or less dismiss her.
- Mr Blue stands on (other residents') feet, Mr Black shouts at him. Mr Blue's dementia has progressed beyond theirs, he can't communicate with them, he stares into walls. They can't understand why he can't see them.

Residents might demand that strangers or intruders left their house, or two people could think that the same handbag was theirs and fight over it. Their perceptions could vary from each other's, and from hour to hour.

Staff interventions and expectations seem to have influenced how people with dementia interacted. Staff said that residents would not talk much if conversation were not lead by them. They also thought they should intervene if anyone was getting emotionally or physically hurt, but that generally falling out with each other is part of everyday life and staff did not always have to step in. Staff could create situations when residents had to interact, for example by expecting that they worked together to set tables and clear dishes.

Staff thought that the ideal group would be a homogeneous one where residents were similar in terms of their type and level of dementia, and their social background. An equal gender mix was thought to make a healthier group. Such an ideal group was in practice very difficult to achieve: dementia progressed in different rates and ways, and more women than men were referred. Staff also thought that there could come a point where group living did not benefit the resident any more, and could upset others too much.

It is very difficult for people without dementia to understand those who are affected. The interviews suggested that we may more easily see the point of view of those least affected, than the perspective of the most disabled.

This qualitative study raised general questions about how people with dementia got on with each other which it was not designed to answer, but which seem important to follow up. Are these patterns of interactions and relationships typical of other pragmatic groups too?

Conclusion: could pragmatic groups be better for people with dementia?

In summary, from my own study and a literature review, I conclude that:

- much more attention needs to be paid to interactions and relationships between people with dementia in pragmatic groups. Recipients are likely to spend considerable amounts of time in each other's company, and so communication and interaction between them will affect their well-being, positively or negatively. Good quality of care must include promoting good relationships and opportunities to interact positively;
- staff have to discuss and agree when and how they should intervene. What can they do to promote good interactions? When does 'healthy assertiveness' become 'aggressive behaviour'? Is this the point where people may be sedated?
- people with dementia may be slower to adjust to new company, but like all of us, they actively judge each other's behaviour and standards. Both residents and staff may find it difficult to tolerate diversity, but on the other hand, diversity might be stimulating;
- those of us without dementia have to be careful not to side with the least affected.

There are no easy answers. Pragmatic groups exist mainly because of lack of resources. Dementia progresses at different rates and in different ways. Increased awareness and discussion of the way that people with dementia relate to each other, however, could help to improve the quality of care offered.

A chapter on this subject can really only raise further questions: What ideally can people with dementia gain from each other's company? Can the disadvantages of pragmatic groups be overcome? Who would people with dementia choose to be with if they could? Is such choice only possible for the wealthy?

Note

1 Their names have been changed.

References

Bleathman C and Morton I (1994) Psychological treatments. In Burns A and Levy R (eds) *Dementia*. London: Chapman and Hall.

Dean R, Proudfoot R and Lindesay J (1993) The Quality of Interactions Schedule (QUIS): development, reliability and use in the evaluation of two domus units. *International Journal. of Geriatric Psychiatry* 8, 819-826.

Holden UP and Woods RT (1995). *Positive Approaches to Dementia Care* (Third Edition). Edinburgh: Churchill Livingstone.

Jones G (1991) A communication model for the care of the elderly. Chapter 6 in Jones G and Miesen BML (eds) *Care-Giving in Dementia: Resarch and Applications*. London: Routledge.

Kitwood T and Bredin K (1992) Towards a theory of dementia care: personhood and well-being. *Ageing and Society* 12 , 269-287.

Levin E, Sinclair I and Gorbach P (1989) *Families, Services and Confusion in Old Age*. London: Avebury

Lubinski R (ed) (1991) *Dementia and Communication*. Philadelphia: BC Decker.

Moos R and Lemke S (1984) *Multiphasic Environmental Assessment Procedure* (MEAP) Manual. Social Ecology Laboratory, Stanford University, Palo Alto, California.

Netten A (1993) *A Positive Environment?* Aldershot: Ashgate.

Wilkin D and Hughes B (1987) Residential care of elderly people: the consumer's views. *Ageing and Society* 7, 175-201.

Willcocks D, Peace S and Kellaher L (1987) *Private Lives in Public Places*. London: Tavistock.

15 Staff issues in the hospital and in the community: a case for retaining longstay hospital provision

Alan Gilloran

Community care as an orthodox approach

It has become increasingly acknowledged that community care is better than institutional care for a wide range of people requiring varying levels of support. Politicians of all hues endorse the principle of care in the community, although they may bicker and score points about issues of resourcing. Further down the command chain policy makers and then practitioners offer similar views, although here the caveats expressed may relate more to disquiet over implementation and the unfortunate warring of professional tribes. Equally in today's 'breeze block towers' academic researchers, while also voicing criticisms, tend mainly to go along with the principles behind community care policies. Thus community care as an idea has taken on the mantle of the orthodox.

Institutional 'care' is now reconceived in terms of incarceration, control or custody and as such immediately registers a negative response. Pointed out early by Barton (1959), then by the more widely read Goffman (1961) and on through work such as Wing and Brown (1970), few can have escaped the growing knowledge that the institutions which we constructed throughout the nineteenth century to care for various segregated groups of people, were in fact places not necessarily serving their best interests. Indeed in policy terms the notion to care for people in community settings was discussed as early as the Royal Commission of 1924-26. Within our current ways of thinking institutional care for people who are elderly or who have mental health difficulties, learning difficulties or physical disabilities has come to represent a last resort and one for which we should be continually searching for alternatives. The care of people with dementia would also fall into this category.

However, before institutions are entirely booed off the stage, like the ubiquitous pantomime baddie, perhaps we should pause and ask certain questions. First, are all institutions bad? Second, are institutions bad for everyone in them? Third, are all the characteristics of institutions bad? If all the answers are confirmed positive then by all means let us be rid of them. However, I would hazard a guess that this will not in fact be the case.

In this short piece I wish to adopt the stance of devil's advocate and begin to build a case for the retention of a longstay hospital sector for people with dementia which should be responded to in a positive manner. For this I shall primarily focus on issues from a staff perspective, although the relationship between this angle and the quality of the care received by people with dementia is plain.

Caring for people with dementia

One of the main reasons for people with dementia being referred to care settings is the recognition by carers that they can no longer cope. Whether it is prompted by the never-ending grind of manual work, such as lifting and washing, or by the distress and feelings of helplessness which challenging behaviour may bring or simply through not knowing what to do, a caregiver may feel the need to seek help. (Interesting recent research by Chappell and Penning (1996) has attempted to identify the specific behaviours which are most associated with distress and feeling burdened on the part of caregivers.)

These same difficulties and challenges, however, are also experienced by staff caring for people with dementia and the work in longstay hospital wards, residential care homes, care housing and nursing homes is known to be both physically and mentally difficult and exhausting.

Staff members who feel run ragged, frustrated or distressed, however, have colleagues with whom they can share their feelings, unwind or discuss difficult issues, as well as having the obvious escape of going home at the end of their shift. I would argue that a crucial point relates to scale in that if we continue to develop units of ever-decreasing size then we may run the risk of subjecting care workers to similar pressures as those experienced by the carers. In other words as the number of people with dementia housed in one place decreases the concomitant number of care staff also diminishes, which in turn reduces significantly the available degree of support for those staff. The size of units for people with dementia has been discussed widely, especially since the Timbury Report (1979), however the focus of concern has primarily been upon residents or patients as opposed to staff. Such an omission needs to be rectified.

From research with members of staff faced with relocation or hospital closure, Ramon (1992) has identified feelings akin to bereavement as they perceive the event as bringing an important part of their life to a close. They are losing security and the comfort of known surroundings but they may also be grieving for the loss of support and friendship which went hand-in-hand with working in the hospital. It may be that staff who transfer to smaller, community-oriented units are able to somehow re-create support networks but at present there is a lack of research attention in this area.

The underlying principle of community care for those in need of support is to maintain independence and to provide care settings which are as homely as possible. Care staff are obviously an important integral part of this process and recent published work has drawn attention to the relationship between levels of work satisfaction and the quality of care received by people with dementia (see Gilloran et al, 1995; Robertson et al, 1995). On the basis of this identified association between higher levels of expressed satisfaction and better observed care quality, close attention consequently requires to be paid to the needs of care staff as well as to the people with dementia. Perhaps the concept of personhood so popular in discussions in the field of dementia care needs to be equally applied to the staff who are involved in the care and support.

An alternative way forward: communities in hospitals

Few would argue that we should leave longstay hospital wards as they are with the lack of a stimulating environment, characterised so often by the image of rows of high-back chairs ringing the day room as if they are attached to the wallpaper. In truth, however, many longstay wards are not like this at all with instead chairs arranged around small tables, small seating areas created in corridor recesses, pictures on the walls and some personal possessions available and on show. Staff in many of the longstay hospital wards throughout Scotland in which I have conducted research have struggled hard to creatively produce a more personalised and homely care setting. In other words certain negative aspects of institutions, such as the lack of a stimulating environment, are being addressed, so that not all of an institution's characteristics may be as detrimental to the interests of people with dementia as was once the case.

In similar ways staff working with the benefit of appropriate facilities and staffing may encourage some people with dementia to make tea/coffee and snacks or go out on visits which again allows movement away from the rigidity of a formally administered round of life, to borrow from Goffman. As identified in recent research (Gilloran et al, 1995) the best care quality in wards for people with dementia is achieved through a relationship between staff who have high levels of job satisfaction and who also enjoy support from management with regard to innovative aspects of care. Good quality care in an institutional setting is therefore achievable although improvements are always possible. It is worth pointing out that even where the physical environment may appear initially unpromising to assume that the care delivered reflects this may actually be spurious and may be injurious to a particularly dedicated group of staff.

Where the institutional environment, as represented by the longstay hospital ward, obviously falls down is in its degree of isolation from the wider community. However, at this point we need to consider that the hospital too represents a community, possibly more so for staff but also for patients. The question then becomes can ways be found to reduce this isolation from the wider society in a manner which will benefit staff in terms of ensuring support networks as well as the people with dementia through continuing to assist in the promotion of independence and in creating a homely environment.

In Scotland a report entitled *Mental Hospitals in Focus* (1989) floated the concept of 'a mental health campus'. This contained the idea of assembling a range of services on one site including in-patient, out-patient and day care. It would therefore seem but a short step to expand this conceptualisation to incorporate certain other provision such as residential units or sheltered accommodation as well as incorporating a range of therapeutic interventions. The report's authors suggested that units for people with dementia might be 'more appropriately sited in isolation from the other units' (1989 para 78) but I cannot agree with this reasoning. I would question the necessity for such a campus to be strictly mental health oriented and indeed there may be good arguments for this not to be the case, for example in reducing stigma and in creating a more multi-faceted environment.

Further to turn community care entirely on its head it could be possible to bring the community into such a broadly 'institutional' setting by breaking down the barriers between hospital and public facilities. Why not have rented or privately owned flats within the hospital or campus grounds with cafes and shops available for all who inhabit that space? The advantages and disadvantages for people who are in receipt of some kind of care would have to be debated but, in keeping with my main concern, staff working in such an environment would benefit through having access to others with a range of experiences who can support them. Not only would staff be available to support each other but the opportunities for learning and development would also be enhanced. We would therefore be creating communities of care rather than expecting the community to care, albeit with the assistance of teams of peripatetic but potentially unconnected professionals.

Conclusion

From a staff perspective I have expressed certain concerns regarding the size of units providing care for people with dementia and I have also suggested that retaining a longstay hospital facility within a reconstituted environment could be beneficial.

The concept of 'home for life' for people with dementia in residential or care housing is a matter which provokes some debate and I would argue that a health campus may provide greater flexibility for individuals to move between the most appropriate and specific care settings. One advantage would be that at least the external locality would still be a known environment for that person as well as for any of their relatives or friends who visit.

Overall my argument is based upon a refutation that all institutions are bad, that they are bad for everyone in them and that all their characteristics act against the interests of those for whom they purport to care. I do not, however, advocate a return to the kind of institutions which were run by staff mafias for those same self-interested groups. Rather I make a plea for the recognition of the positive aspects of working in longstay hospital settings which may be all too easily lost in the rhetoric of community care and the perceived need to malign a previous approach to care. Let us therefore not forget the needs of care staff who are increasingly being reallocated to work in community settings often experiencing a lack of role clarity and uncertainty over sources of support. Under such circumstances expecting an improvement in the quality of care in comparison with that delivered in longstay wards may be misplaced.

References

Barton WR (1959) *Institutional Neurosis*. Bristol: Wright & Sons.

Chappell NL and Penning M (1996) Behavioural problems and distress among caregivers of people with dementia. *Ageing and Society* 16, 57-73.

Gilloran A, Robertson A, McGlew T and McKee K (1995) Improving work satisfaction amongst nursing staff and the quality of care for elderly patients with dementia: some policy implications. *Ageing and Society* 15, 375-391.

Goffman E (1961) *Asylums*. Harmondsworth: Penguin.

Mental Hospitals in Focus (1989) *Report by a Working Group of NMCC on the Future Role of Mental Illness Hospitals in Scotland*. Edinburgh: HMSO.

Ramon S (1992) Being at the receiving end of the closure process. In Ramon S (ed) *Psychiatric Hospital Closure*. London: Chapman and Hall.

Robertson A, Gilloran A, McGlew T, McKee K, McKinley A and Wight D (1995) Nurses job satisfaction and the quality of care received by patients in psychogeriatric wards. *International Journal of Geriatric Psychiatry* 10, 575-584.

Royal Commission on Lunacy and Mental Disorder (1924-26) Macmillan Commission.

Timbury Report (1979) *Report on Services for the Elderly with Mental Disability in Scotland*. Edinburgh: HMSO.

Wing JK and Brown G (1970) *Institutionalism and Schizophrenia*. Cambridge University Press.

16 Problems in recognising dementia in general practice: how can they be overcome?

Steve Iliffe

The early signs of dementia are often missed by family members and professionals alike, and both groups may do little in response to the growing symptoms of dementia. This may not matter, as long as family members and professionals remain equally unaware. For example, interviews with the relatives of predominantly working class elderly people with early dementia in Cambridge (Pollitt et al, 1989) suggested that most did not view the changes in their dementing relative as a matter of serious concern, and saw loss of daily living skills as part of normal ageing rather than as a symptom of illness. In the majority of instances the changes in the affected individual had not been brought to the attention of their family doctor, possibly because of different social class attitudes to the role of the general practitioner, with middle class families having a more social and less narrowly medical perception of general practitioners functions (Ineichen, 1994)

A similar study of relatives of elderly Italian people in whom a diagnosis of dementia had been reached during a hospital admission for an unrelated problem found three main reasons for delayed diagnosis: attribution of change to normal ageing; respect for parents or grandparents; and negligible effect of the problem on family life and the family economy (Antonelli Incalzi et al, 1992) Even older people who have frequent contact with general practitioners may not report symptoms of forgetfulness or confusion. A community study in East London found only a minority of those aged 85 and over (with an annual consultation rate of seven) had consulted their general practitioner about memory or cognitive changes, although one in three experienced forgetfulness and one in six experienced confusion (Bowling, 1989)

If the early signs of dementia cause no major problems for those around the individual whose cognitive function and everyday abilities are deteriorating, a diagnosis of dementia is not needed, and is not made. We know that failure to diagnose dementia by general practitioners is common if medical records are compared with the results of population screening for cognitive impairment (Iliffe et al, 1991), and the diagnosis may be absent from the medical records of individuals with very advanced dementia. Some obstacle to documenting (rather than making) a diagnosis seems to operate, because the ability of general practitioners to reach a diagnosis of dementia when prompted about particular cases in experimental studies is better than might be expected (O'Connor et al, 1988), especially if guidelines for diagnosis are used (Cooper et al, 1992). While some of the failure to document the diagnosis may reflect hurried and inconsistent record-keeping, anecdotal evidence from carers and families suggests that there is also a real problem of recognition in everyday practice. Part of this problem of delayed diagnosis appears to lie with the clinician's own emotional response to the diagnosis, and part with a limited conceptual framework for understanding dementia.

Interviews with Belgian general practitioners about their patients with dementia (De Lepeleire et al, 1994) revealed that doctors (and patients) initially denied problems created by the dementing process, began the diagnostic process when the patient became a significant problem to others, and responded to the diagnosis – once made – with feelings of disbelief, of apprehension at the level of support that the family would require, of frustration at their own powerlessness, and of fear of dementia itself. A similar process of being paralysed or overwhelmed by the complexities of the situation is described amongst nurses working with older people (Whall, 1992)

Diagnostic triggers

A number of factors triggered the diagnosis of dementia amongst the Belgian general practitioners:

- disturbances in activities of daily living, including irregularities in medication usage in individuals who had previously been reliable in their use of prescribed medicines for long-term problems;
- behavioural problems like expression of and action around paranoid ideas or hallucinations, which cause major problems for family and neighbours;
- cognitive disturbances, with memory loss or orientation difficulties, so that bills are not paid, important things mislaid or the individuals themselves becoming lost in familiar environments;
- crises – 'revelatory moments' – like the sudden loss of support from a spouse who becomes acutely ill and is admitted to hospital, or an intercurrent illness in the dementia sufferer themselves, which adds acute confusion to the underlying but camouflaged chronic confusional state.

These diagnostic triggers and revelatory moments may result in urgent referrals to specialist services that may be perceived by other professionals as being 'too late' (Ineichen, 1994), but can they be avoided by earlier diagnosis and more timely intervention within primary care?

Good practice

Since general practice is a discipline that solves problems, rather than reaches diagnoses, early detection of and earlier responses to dementia may not be feasible as long as the changes of dementia are contained within a family or social structure and wrongly attributed to normal ageing. However, we know from experience that there is sufficient mismatch between family perceptions and professional judgements about individuals with symptoms of dementia to justify a more critical perspective, and warrant investment of time and effort in promoting 'good practice' in the recognition of dementia, and in making responses to it. Four issues appear important in the development of such 'good practice' in primary care: a population perspective on health care in later life; enhancement of diagnostic skills; application of the continuing care paradigm to dementia; and networking with appropriate social, voluntary and medical agencies.

Population perspective
The current general practitioner contract requires all GPs to offer all their patients aged 75 and over an annual assessment of their health, in their home, including an assessment of their 'mental condition'. This contractual obligation

is widely unpopular in general practice, is often ignored or performed perfunctorily, and where done may be delegated to other practice staff. However, it does allow a profile of the older population to be created and permits a systematic review of mental health, and this may allow earlier detection of unrecognised dementia and permit forward planning to minimise the impact of crises. If it is to be widely and effectively applied it will have to be seen as useful for patients and professionals alike, and this will require investment in training for primary care staff.

Enhanced diagnostic skills
The tendency to misdiagnose individuals with physical frailty and functional psychiatric disorders as demented has been noted by Philp (Philp and Young, 1988) and may explain the tendency of general practitioners to over-diagnose the condition when prompted on a case-by-case basis (Cooper, 1992; O'Connor, 1988). None of the general practitioners in the Belgian study could give an operational definition of, or accepted diagnostic criteria for, dementia (De Lepeleire, 1994). Nor did they include depression when discussing alternative diagnoses, but they did describe four of the key symptoms in the DSMIIIR criteria – ADL disturbance, behaviour change, memory loss and disorientation – and emphasised the importance of the clinical picture and of informant histories.

Validated screening instruments, used either in population screening or in clinical encounters, appear to offer an alternative to enhanced clinical skills, but they are not widely used in general practice. In a study of general practitioners in Edinburgh only 14 per cent used a standard cognitive function test (MacKenzie, 1992), while a second and wider survey found less than a quarter using such a test (Barker et al, 1992). Training other staff to use a standard instrument as a screening tool is possible (Iliffe et al, 1990) and may be a useful addition to the 75 and over screening process. However, when general practitioners do use a standard instrument for detecting cognitive impairment on an opportunistic basis as a case-finding tool (in a randomised controlled trial) their subsequent management and referral behaviour does not change (Iliffe et al, 1994).

A broader educational approach emphasising the complexity of the clinical picture in dementia, its evolution over time, the importance of informant histories and the opportunities for useful responses may be more important than reliance on screening tests, and this approach has informed the production of a recent educational package (Alzheimer's Disease Society, 1995).

Dementia and its emotional context
Broad educational approaches may not be helpful unless primary care professionals perceive the dementias as progressive neurological disorders

that cannot be cured, but for which a range of supportive responses still exists. The view that 'nothing can be done' for advanced cancer would not be accepted today, because so many options exist for relieving symptoms and helping the patient and others to overcome the problems of the disease. The same repertoire of responses is needed to overcome the therapeutic nihilism that dementia still provokes. Management strategies for medical, nursing and social care workers will be accepted in primary care if they are seen to 'work' – that is, relieve the patient's distress, reduce the burden on carers, restore a sense of effectiveness to professionals and whenever possible, avoid crises. Including advanced dementia as a condition suitable for a 'continuing' care approach would signal such a change of perception.

Networking

Membership of a local network of services focused on early detection and support of people with dementia and their carers, and rapid response at times of crisis, seems essential if general practitioners are to optimise the care they give. Routes into such networks will vary, but old age psychiatrists may be in a good position to promote networking, for example, by promoting attachment of community psychiatric nurses (CPN) to practices where they have been shown to provide high quality supportive care to people with dementia and their families as well as facilitating early diagnosis (Ineichen, 1994). Social service involvement is essential, but given the culture gap between social work and general practice and the limited resources available to social service departments, it is perhaps the most problematic of all the tasks involved in network development. Nevertheless innovative collaborative work around the needs of older people, particularly those with the kinds of complex needs that people with dementia experience, is developing and a research and development agenda to promote it has been proposed (Dickie and Iliffe, 1996).

Conclusions

A general practitioner or practice nurse who recognises the early symptoms of dementia in a patient, but who then finds that the family do not perceive any serious change, may be tempted to ignore their own knowledge and not document their findings. This is no longer justifiable, in my view, because the suspicion of dementia will alter future consultations, cast urgent requests for assistance by family or neighbours in a different light, allow mobilisation of resources to be thought about in advance – even planned – and prepare primary care workers for discussion of diagnoses and responses when events reveal dementia as a problem. Initial suspicions may be wrong, of course, but they can be reviewed and checked by other team members only if they are recorded. That process of reviewing presupposes a proactive approach to the problem of dementia amongst professionals who are expanding their knowledge base and repertoire of responses to a problem that will neither go away, nor stay hidden for long. We have plenty to do.

References

Alzheimer's Disease Society (1995) *Dementia in the Community: Management Strategies for General Practice*. London: ADS.

Antonelli Incalzi R et al (1992) Unrecognised dementia: sociodemographic correlates. *Aging* (Milano) 4, 327-32.

Barker A et al (1992) Health checks for people over 75. *British Medical Journal* 305, 1098-1099.

Bowling A (1989) Contact with general practitioners and differences in health among people aged over 85 years. *Journal of the Royal College of General Practicioners* 39, 52-55.

Cooper B et al (1992) The ability of general practitioners to detect dementia and cognitive impairment in their elderly patients: a study in Mannheim. *International Journal of Geriatric Psychiatry* 7, 591-8.

De Lepeleire J A et al (1994) How do general practitioners diagnose dementia? *Family Practice* 11, 148-152.

Dickie S and Iliffe S (1996) Bridging the gap between social services and primary care. *British Journal of Health Care Management* 2(5), 258-262.

Iliffe S et al (1990) Screening for cognitive impairment in the elderly using the mini-mental state examination. *British Journal of General Practitioners* 40, 277-279.

Iliffe S et al (1991) Assessment of elderly people in general practice. 1. Social circumstances and mental state. *British Journal of General Practice* 41, 9-12.

Iliffe S et al (1994) Evaluation of the use of brief screening instruments for dementia, depression and problem drinking among elderly people in general practice. *British Journal of General Practitioners* 44, 503-507.

Ineichen B (1994) Managing demented older people in the community: a review. *Family Practice* 11, 210-215.

MacKenzie D M (1992) Screening the mental state of the over 75s in the community: what are GPs doing? *Psychiatry Bulletin* 16, 146-7.

O Connor D W et al (1988) Do general practitioners miss dementia in elderly patients? *British Medical Journal* 297, 1107-1110.

Philp I and Young J (1988) An audit of a primary care teams knowledge of the existence of symptomatic demented elderly. *Health Bulletin* 46, 93-97.

Pollitt B et al (1989) Mild dementia: perception and problems. *Ageing and Society* 9, 261-275.

Whall A L (1992) The problem of missed psychiatric diagnoses in the elderly. *Journal of Gerontological Nursing* 18, 41-42.

17 Old age psychiatry and dementia: somebody cares

David Jolley

Origins

Specialist services for older people with psychiatric disorders began to appear in the United Kingdom during the late 1960s (Jolley and Arie, 1978 and 1992). They followed on from the development of specialist (Geriatric) services for older people whose problems included physical deterioration and dependency (Isaacs, 1981). Both owed their origins to the increase in absolute and relative numbers of people surviving into old age, the prevalence and nature of health problems within late life and the personal and national costs associated with them. While medicine, as a whole, had become intoxicated with its potential to 'cure' illnesses which had hitherto been crippling, debilitating or lethal, old age continued to present problems of 'deterioration', dependency or disturbance which defied all curative powers. Though these characteristics might be deemed the product of multiple pathologies of differing time courses, there was one condition influential above all others and spanning the orbits of physical medicine and psychiatry – this was dementia. Despite all attempts to alter it by manoeuvres of nomenclature and enthusiasms for curative breakthroughs, it remains true to this image.

Essentials

What was needed was a response which accepted the numbers and the characteristics of the condition and said:

> We're here to help and we'll see you through. We don't offer a cure. but we do promise understanding and shared knowledge which can alleviate the worst of the suffering for patients and those (usually their family) who care for them. Throughout we'll bring the best of known medical practice to bear on your difficulties, attending to anything which is treatable, bringing in other experts as necessary and liaising with other agencies who may have better or greater resources to deal with particular aspects or particular phases of the illness.

This was what was needed and this is what the pioneer old age psychiatrists began to provide and began to teach others to do (Arie, 1970).

The first essential was to offer a specialist service happy to see patients who may be suffering from dementia. To be available, to encourage easy referral, often visiting patients at home to make an initial assessment and to begin the process of reassurance, encouragement and commitment which might need to endure for years. This was a massive change in approach from previous tentative postures which saw dementia as untouchable, unworthy of the precious skills of psychiatrists and their teams (Smith, 1961). It also dared to disassociate the expertise of professionals from the back-up of resources under their immediate control (Arie and Jolley, 1982).

Old age psychiatry has not usually restricted its interests and responsibility to dementia but accepts a full range of psychiatric disorders in late life (Jolley et al, 1996). There is a lobby which would argue for specialist services which work only with dementia sufferers and their families. The strength of such an arrangement would seem to be a clear focus without the distraction of calls from other patients with other conditions. This leaves all resources identified for use within the dementia population and encourages all efforts to be concentrated on improving practice in this demanding arena. Yet few services have proved comfortable or sustainable with such a restricted remit.

Maintaining morale within the specialist team is one consideration. In addition the range of skills needed to effect best management of dementia require experience of work with patients suffering from depression, paranoid states and other disorders. While dementia is the core condition of old age psychiatry, older patients with other disorders have always been at risk of neglect, misdiagnosis and misinformation and would be disadvantaged if not included. Indeed the group who have benefited least from the initiatives of the past thirty years is made up of 'graduates' with long established psychoses (Campbell, 1991). Neither should early onset of dementia ('Pre-Senile') be excluded from the benefits of acceptance by old age psychiatry. There have been recurring calls for super specialist services for younger dementia sufferers and their families. The arguments are that the clinical, genetic and social associations of dementia in the pre-senile are different from dementia in very late life and that patients and families are uncomfortable and distressed when a deranged father of 62 years is cared for alongside a majority of women who are over 85 years in age (Alzheimer's Disease Society, 1992).

There is little doubt that where super specialist services have been set up they have been well received and provide excellent care of all sorts and a useful base for research into the special problems on this subset of dementia. Yet it has often proved difficult to accrue resources for such a rare condition requiring a successful project to attract sponsorship from a number of health districts. My own view has shifted from desperation and despair at the failure to create such specialised resources within Greater Manchester, to increasing confidence that where good and reasonably well resourced old age psychiatry services integrate with other interested services, including neurologists, a robust and acceptable compromise can be achieved. The key, as ever, is to say 'yes', and do your best with what you have got, and improve step-wise from there.

Assessment

Assessment is designed to achieve an understanding of the individual and is, therefore, much helped by time spent with the patient and his/her family, preferably in their own home. For it is important to discover the history of genetics, family life, upbringing and later experiences which have combined to produce the present. That history and this present will influence what can be the best and most carefully tended future. More detailed and specific investigations and collations may be undertaken at a clinic or hospital out-patient department, and their findings will enrich and inform the process.

Physical treatments may be available to correct or alleviate an underlying or associated condition or to help control symptoms such as anxiety, sleeplessness, restlessness, or paranoid ideation. Psychotherapeutic approaches to individuals, families and wider groups provide the backbone of good practice.

Seeing it through

Belonging is a powerful tool for dealing with difficulties: 'Once you are with us you need never feel alone', is the message to be conveyed. Holding on tight, but gently, reduces damage and will achieve best use of all the resources. Service registers should be encouraged as a framework for ensuring the best care of people with dementia (Jolley, 1979) and copied to improve care in similar circumstances.

Relationships

Introduction to specialist services may be self-referral (Herzberg, 1995), but is more usually through primary health care or other specialist hospital services (Arie and Jolley, 1996). GPs often know their patients very well (Iliffe et al, 1991; SMOAPS, 1996) and are pleased when specialist services show interest in them and will share actively in their case and follow up care.

Other hospital specialists: orthopaedic surgery, genito-urinary surgery and general medicine are called upon to treat patients with dementia who develop other illnesses or injuries. These are precarious times for patients, and patients families are guarded in their comments on care received. It is not easy to find the best way to serve confused patients within the same ward as others who are not so compromised. Old age psychiatry services rarely do enough to help these situations

More consistently well developed is the relationship with providers of 'social' care at home, or through day centres and various grades of resident-ial/nursing home care (Jolley, 1981). In parts of the United Kingdom very impressive systems are now in place which enable people to live at home, all be it at some risk and at considerable cost, for most of their life with dementia.

Advocacy

Old age psychiatry has played a role in arguing for the advantage of a full and properly balanced range of services for people with dementia. The hardest battle has been to retain or regain an element of specialist terminal (longstay) hospital care for these patients so seriously damaged or disturbed by the condition that they cannot be well managed elsewhere (Jolley, 1994a).

In most instances it has been best to replace mental hospital accommodation with smaller nursing home/community hospital units linked into community services. They function as a resource for education and support of other residential establishments as well as offering direct care to the few patients in greatest need (Jolley, 1994b). There remains a great deal to be learned about practice in the care of patients at home, the best use of day care and respite care and the management of people in care and in the period immediately prior to death (Black and Jolley, 1990).

Basic research

But what of cure? What of a better understanding of the biological basis of the dementia? Has old age psychiatry played a part here and has it a potential for the future of such endeavour? The Newcastle Pioneers (Kay et al, 1964) interwove their research and service activities. Newcastle also produced the first great relationship between clinician (Gary Blessed) and neuropathologist (Bernard Tomlinson) and later Elaine Perry. Alistair Burns (Burns et al, 1990 and 1991) has founded a career on the same approach. Careful clinical analysis linked to new histopathological staining techniques, in both Newcastle and Nottingham, revealed Lewy Body dementia as a new syndrome differing in aetiology, clinical features outcome and response to medication. Clinicians have played a part in bringing families with strong histories of illness into contact with geneticists who have identified specific chromosomal abnormalities in some familial dementias. And clinicians are exercised to evaluate the advantages and hazards of new therapies.

Mainline

The most important contribution of old age psychiatry to the history of dementia has been that it has provided a home for sufferers and carers and a system of organisation within the range of services that says: 'You belong here'. Within this security all else is proving possible and despair is set aside.

References

Alzheimer's Disease Society (1992) *The Younger Person with Dementia*. London: ADS.

Arie T (1970). The first year of the Goodmayes psychiatric service for old people. *Lancet* 2, 1179-1182.

Arie T and Jolley D (1982). Making services work: organisation and style of psychogeriatric services. In Levy R and Post F (eds) *The Psychiatry of Late Life*. Oxford: Blackwell Scientific, 222-251.

Arie T and Jolley D (1996) Psychogeriatric Care. Chapter 42 in Tallis R and Brocklehurst J (eds) *Textbook of Geriatric Medicine and Gerontology 5*. Edinburgh: Churchill Livingstone.

Black D and Jolley D (1990) Slow euthanasia? The deaths of psychogeriatric patients. *British Medical Journal* 300, 1321-1323.

Burns A, Lewis G, Jacoby R and Levy R (1991) Factors affecting survival in Alzheimer's Disease. *Psychological Medicine* 21(2), 363-370.

Burns A, Cuthbert P, Levy R, Jacoby J and Lantos P (1990) Accuracy of clinical diagnosis in Alzheimer's Disease. *British Medical Journal* 301, 1026.

Campbell P (1991) Graduates. Chapter 22 in Jacoby R and Oppenheimer C (eds) *Psychiatry in the Elderly*. Oxford Medical Publications.

Herzberg J (1995). Can multidisciplinary teams carry out competent and safe psychogeriatric assessments in the community? *International Journal of Geriatric Psychiatry* 10, 173-177.

Iliffe S, Haines A and Gallivan S (1991) Assessment of elderly people in general practice. 1. Social circumstances and mental state. *British Journal of General Practice* 41, 9-12.

Isaacs B (1981) Is Geriatrics a Specialty? Chapter 14 in Arie T (ed) *Health Care of the Elderly*. London: Croom Helm, 224-235.

Jolley D (1979) All is not lost. In Molly Meacher (ed) *New Approaches to the Management of Old People with Mental Health Problems in Continuing Care Settings*. London: Mental Health Foundation/ Pergamon Press, 195-207.

Jolley D (1981) Misfits in need of care. Chapter 5 in Arie T (ed) *Health Care of the Elderly*. London: Croom Helm, 71-88.

Jolley D (1994a) The future of long-stay care as a public health provision. *Reviews in Clinical Gerontology* 4, 1-4.

Jolley D (1994b) Independent means. *Care of the Elderly*, October, 373-376.

Jolley D and Arie T (1978) The organisation of psychogeriatric services. *British Journal of Psychiatry* 132, 1-11.

Jolley D and Arie T (1992). Developments in psychogeriatric services. In Arie T (ed) *Recent Advances in Psychogeriatrics* no 2. Edinburgh: Churchill Livingstone, 117-135.

Jolley D, Russell E and Lennon S (1996) The organisation of services in Old Age Psychiatry: a review of the present state of things. Chapter in Pathy MSJ (ed) *Principles and Practice of Geriatric Medicine* (third edition). Chichester: John Wiley.

Kay DWK, Beamish P and Roth M (1964a) Old age mental disorders in Newcastle upon Tyne: Part 1: A study of prevalence. *British Journal of Psychiatry* 110, 146-158.

Kay DWK, Beamish P and Roth M (1964b) Old age mental disorders in Newcastle upon Tyne: Part 2: A study of possible social and medical causes. *British Journal of Psychiatry*.

Kay DWK, Bergmann K, Foster EM, McKechnie AA and Roth M (1970) Mental illness and hospital usage in the elderly. *Comprehensive Psychiatry* 1, 26-35.

Smith S (1961) Psychiatry in general hospitals. *Lancet* (ii), 1158-1159.

South Manchester Old Age Psychiatry Service (SMOAPS) (1996) Interviews with General Practitioners. *Survey of mental health of old people in South Manchester*. Local report.

18 Group homes: an alternative for older people with dementia

Bo Malmberg

In the 1960s and 1970s there was, especially when looking back on the situation, almost unlimited scope for public sector activities in Sweden. This applied not least to the elderly and the expansion of old age care. The home help services markedly increased during these decades and in 1975 almost 40 per cent of all Swedes aged 80 and more had some kind of home help. This figure is now down to below 25 per cent (Malmberg and Sundström, 1996).

As the provision of home help peaked, it became more and more difficult to provide satisfactory home help care to persons suffering from dementia and this remains the case today. People with moderate to severe dementia, who have home help, soon have to move to an institution even if relatives are prepared to give a lot of support in the home (Sundström et al, 1994). In an ongoing study of old age care in the county of Jönköping, among other things all institutions for the elderly are being investigated. In a study of more than 5,200 people who live in any kind of old age institution in the county, it was found that only about one-third are mentally quite alert according to the Berger rating of the severity of senility scale (Berger, 1980). This means that two-thirds have some kind of mental confusion, often only disruptive forgetfulness (almost one-fifth), but half of the people have more severe mental problems. The concentration of people not quite mentally alert at the old age institutions points to the problems the home help service has taking care of them at home. It is tragic that those people who often would have gained most staying in a well-known environment are the same people that the home help service and/or the family find the most difficult to help in their homes.

To relieve the home help service and to help relatives take care of the demented living at home, day care centres for people with dementia were introduced in the late 1970s and 1980s. Nowadays most Swedish municipalities have this kind of facility and it is estimated that about 12,000 people are taking part in the programme offered by the day care centres for the demented in Sweden (Hansson et al, 1996).

Day care centres usually cater for eight to twelve people. Patients will often make up two groups, each group attending every second day. Roughly, therefore, each programme serves about twenty people. As well as relieving the home help service and relatives, the centres aim to provide a meaningful day for the participants, keeping them as active as possible with everyday tasks, indoors and outdoors. The activities are done together with the centre staff who act as role models. Much of the activities are tied to the meals that are offered at the day care centres. The personnel prepare food, lay the table, eat and do the dishes together with the clients. This means a close and intense relationship develops between the staff and the person with dementia. The staff usually attend special introductory courses to prepare for this close contact. However, despite the staff's efforts the drop-out rate in the programmes is rather high. In a year almost half of the clients ceased to participate, one evaluation has shown (Malmberg and Oremark, 1989). The alternative then is often to move the person with dementia to some kind of institution.

At the end of the 1970s in Sweden a good alternative to existing institutional care was lacking for older people with dementia. The Swedish Board of Social Welfare recommended that they should be integrated in the established old age care institutions, particularly in the nursing homes. But the staff often thought that dementia sufferers did not 'fit in' there, or where ever they lived for that matter (Hedvall and Johansson, 1983).

At the beginning of the 1980s group homes were introduced on a small scale. This was the first, and is still the only, institution in Sweden to have been directly designed to meet the needs of the elderly demented person. The group homes were usually built as small units comprising six to eight small flats clustered around a shared kitchen and living room. The residents live in their own accommodation with tenancy contracts for their flats, and care staff are available 24 hours a day. Residents bring their own furniture, curtains, pictures for the walls and other decorations. The common areas are often furnished with rather old-fashioned furniture that the staff, sometimes together with a resident, have bought at an auction or at a flea market. Taking into account the experiences of the day care programme, the aim is to provide dementia sufferers with a form of accommodation characterised by a home environment and participation in everyday activities. The secondary problems associated with dementia, such as depression, restlessness and anxiety are thought to be reduced by the homely environment and the active participation of the staff as social role models.

Thanks to government money earmarked especially there has been a rapid growth in the number of group homes. While there were only one or two group homes in the early 1980s, the number has risen to around sixty group homes for some 500 pensioners in 1987. In 1992 some 5,300 people were living in group homes and in 1994 just over 14,000 were doing so, according to an evaluation carried out that year (Socialstyrelsen, 1995). The number for 1994 is obviously exaggerated by the tendency to classify institutions as group homes. For example almost 2,000 people who live in what the local authorities call group homes do not even have their own room. There has been some debate about the risk of making the concept of a group home a nonsense. Still, many elderly people with dementia in Sweden now have the opportunity to live in the more original type of group home.

Residents are referred to the group homes by community help teams which coordinate care for elderly people living in the community. Group homes are considered to be an alternative primarily for people that have a moderately severe dementia. It is possible to provide care to persons with milder dementia in their homes and those with more severe dementia are not thought to gain anything from living in a group home. When someone is identified as a possible resident for an available apartment, in the ideal case a member of staff goes to visit the potential resident. Severely demented, very aggressive or agitated people will be directed to nursing homes, instead of group homes. The reason for this is that the nursing homes have more personnel in general and, particularly, more trained medical personnel.

As was reported some years ago (Malmberg and Oremark, 1991; Malmberg and Zarit, 1993) an evaluation of the first four group homes in Jönköping showed that the group homes provide a very calm, non-institutional environment. Residents' apartments are filled with their furniture, photos, pictures and other memorabilia. The common areas have been furnished with ordinary furniture that contributes to the home-like setting. Residents are generally calm and there are seldom problems with aggression and disruptive behavior. This can reflect the initial selection but as the dementia is progressive it is also possible that the environment itself may reduce behaviour problems.

After one year, 36 of the original 40 residents still lived there. Two had died at the group home and although this was a difficult time for the personnel they felt that this was a natural process, and they were proud that the resident did not have to move to a hospital during their final illness. The other two, however, had to be moved to other facilities because of behaviour problems that could not be handled. The people that remained in the group home were rated by the staff to have stable or declining mental functions after one year, but improved behaviour and mood.

The relatives and staff were interviewed after one year. The relatives were very positive about the group home idea. They were most concerned about the staff and how they would cope in the long run. Clearly there are risks of burn-out working so closely with the residents who have a progressive illness. The group home staff were very positive in ratings of their co-workers but also reported some stress; the signs of breakdown were few. The staff feel that this is the right way to work with these clients. For many of them the work is also a great source of satisfaction and even pride. The major problem reported by the staff was that the residents were more demented than they had thought. It was difficult to motivate residents to take part in activities. Because of the diversity in motivation and capacity, staff did more one-to-one than group activities.

The staff are ambivalent towards the resident staying on at the group home when their illness progresses. They want them to stay as they realise that it is upsetting and difficult for the demented to move, and that there is no really good alternative for them. At the same time they realise that some residents have to leave because the staff cannot handle their problems, especially if they become aggressive or show disruptive behaviour by, for example, constantly screaming.

Malmberg and Zarit (1993) also conducted a follow-up study on the original residents after four years for two of the homes and five years for the other two. Of the original 40 residents, 12 still lived in the group homes, 10 had died there, and 18 had been moved to another facility. Retrospective accounts suggested that most relocations were due to declining health and mobility, while a smaller number were because of difficulties managing the resident in the group home. In a four year follow-up study of 16 patients with dementia that initially lived at a group home, Wimo et al (1995) report that aggression was the most frequent reason for leaving the group home for another institution.

So the social approach that is a characteristic of the group home does have its drawbacks. The idea works very well if no serious disruptive behaviour emerges in the progression of the dementia. However, when it does we lack good gero-psychiatric expertise to cooperate with the group home staff without disturbing the social approach, and we lack an institution specially designed for the elderly demented where a medical-psychiatric approach can work side by side with the social one.

References

Berger EY (1980) A system for rating the severity of senility. *Journal of the American Geriatric Society* 28, 234-236.

Hansson JH, Samuelsson L and Berg S (1996) *Dagverksamheter för äldre: En nationell kartläggning (Day Care Facilities for Elderly: A Nationwide Exploration).* Socialstyrelsen, édelutvårderingen 95, 12.

Hedvall R and Johansson L (1983) Några reflektioner kring omhändertagande av åldersdementa *(Some Reflections of the Care-Taking of Demented in Old Age).* *Socialmedicinsk Tidskrift* 60, 545-549.

Malmberg B and Oremark I (1989) *Dagvård för personer med åldersdement beteende (Day Care for Persons with Demented Behavior in Old Age).* Jönköping: Institutet för Gerontologi, Rapport nr 67.

Malmberg B and Oremark I (1991) *En utvärdering av fyra gruppboenden för åldersdementa i Jönköping (An Evaluation of Four Group Homes for Demented in Old Age in Jönköping).* Jönköping: Institutet för gerontologi, Rapport nr 72.

Malmberg B and Sundström G (1996) *Age care crisis in Sweden?* Current Sweden no 412. Stockholm: The Swedish Institute.

Malmberg B and Zarit SH (1993) Group homes for people with dementia: a Swedish example. *Gerontologist* 33, 682-686.

Sundström G, Larsson B and Sjöstrand P (1994) *Hemtjänst före och efter Ädel (Home Help Services before and after Reforms of Old Age Care).* Stockholm: Socialstyrelsen, Ädelutvärderingen 94, 7.

Wimo A, Asplund K, Mattsson B, Adolfsson R and Lundgren K (1995) Patients with dementia in group living: experiences 4 years after admission. *International Psychogeriatrics* 7, 123-127.

19 Personal finances and elderly people with dementia: a challenge for local authorities

Robin Means

Introduction

The community care changes brought in by the NHS and Community Care Act 1990 have had the effect of massively extending the role of local authorities in personal finance issues relating to older people. For example, they are now heavily involved in assessing elderly people for charges relating to nursing home care, residential care and domiciliary services.

The focus of this chapter is not only upon the challenge faced by local authorities in terms of making such charging systems 'work' when the client has dementia, but also more generally in terms of their obligations to protect elderly service users from financial exploitation.

Handling the money of elderly people with dementia

The starting point to explore these issues is to profile the main options in England and Wales for handling the personal finances of an elderly person with dementia (see Figure 19.1). If the person is on benefit, the Benefits Agency needs to be approached and the appropriate appointeeship form filled out. Appointees are responsible to the Secretary of State for using the benefit in the best interests of the claimant who lacks capacity. The vast majority of appointees are relatives, but this role can also be performed by friends, solicitors, local authorities and more controversially by the proprietors of residential and nursing homes.

When the person with dementia has considerable resources, there are four main possibilities. First, building societies and banks will sometimes allow a third person, usually a relative, access to their accounts on an informal basis. Second, people can take out an enduring power of attorney (EPA) when they still have capacity. An EPA can take effect immediately or be drawn up so that it takes effect from the onset of dementia. In either case, the EPA must be registered with the Court of Protection, once dementia has been diagnosed.

Figure 19.1 Handling the money of a person with mental incapacity: administrative and legal options

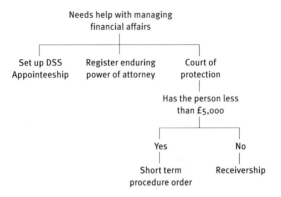

The final two options, receivership and short procedure orders can be applied for through the Court of Protection on behalf of mentally incapacitated adults who have not taken out an enduring power of attorney. Receivership is usually instituted when assets exceed £5,000 and short procedure orders when assets are less. The National Audit Office (1994) examination of this system found 30,000 patients with assets of £780 million. Only 2 per cent of these were on short procedure orders, while receivers were spread between relatives and friends (68 per cent), professionals such as solicitors (9 per cent) and local authorities (2 per cent).

The general view is that this legal and administrative framework is not only confusing, cumbersome and costly, but also lacks sufficient safeguards for the person who lacks capacity (Law Commission, 1995; Langan and Means, 1995; Age Concern, 1996). What are the implications of this for local authorities in the context of the new community care?

Personal finances, elderly people with dementia and local authorities: the research evidence

Langan and Means (1995) carried out a detailed study of the charging policies of three local authorities; a telephone survey of twenty-seven local authorities about their approach to appointeeship and receivership issues; and focus group interviews with thirty-seven field-level staff about their work concerns in the general area of personal finances and elderly people with dementia. Findings suggested local authorities were struggling to respond adequately on a number of fronts.

Charging systems and elderly people with dementia
The charging systems in the three local authorities were varied especially in terms of approaches to charging for home care and other domiciliary services. They were also complex and confusing from the point of view of the service user and carer, and characterised by conflict between social workers/care managers who carried out the assessment and finance/revenue staff who assessed the charge. Under these circumstances, it was perhaps not surprising that no clear advice was available to staff on the 'dos' and 'don'ts' of carrying out an assessment where the service user is known or believed likely to have dementia. In practice, it was clear that an enormous reliance was placed upon information supplied by relatives and friends.

Only one of the three local authorities provided assessment staff with clear information on appointeeship, enduring power of attorney, short procedure orders and receivership and the circumstances under which the local authority might consider taking on appointeeship or receivership roles. All three allowed residential and nursing home proprietors to be appointees; guidance to staff on access to personal finances where the new resident lacked mental capacity was often limited; and no detailed guidance existed for home care and other domiciliary staff about money handling issues which are bound to arise when providing a service for an elderly person with dementia in their own home.

The local authority as appointee or receiver
Both the telephone survey of twenty-seven local authorities and the three case studies identified considerable variation in the attitudes and approaches of local authorities towards taking on appointeeship and receivership roles. In terms of receivership, there were numerous variations in the volume of such work, the designated receiver (director of finance, director of social services etc) and the location of receivership work (most commonly in finance sections). The willingness to take on this role seemed to have emerged from a desire to ensure fee collection for those in local authority residential care. Local authorities were only now beginning to recognise the responsibility of the receiver to act in the best interests of the elderly person, and the implications of this for the location, line management and job description of people carrying out receivership work.

Variation was even greater over appointeeship. Individual authorities often took different stances according to whether the elderly person was in local authority residential care, independent sector care or living at home with a care package. Several authorities were keenest to take on appointeeship roles for those in their own residential care, which again suggests policies being driven by a desire to ease fee collection rather than to protect vulnerable adults. The situation was extremely unclear for elderly people in the community in most local authorities with area offices sometimes pursuing different approaches and with local authorities often lacking a clear picture of the overall number of their appointeeships.

Unsupported field-level staff
The focus group interviews with field-level staff (home care organisers, home care assistants, care managers, etc) underlined the 'knock on' consequences for staff in day-to-day contact with clients of the broad failure of local authorities to develop clear policies on personal finance issues and elderly people with dementia.

This can be illustrated by three examples. First, staff indicated that they felt there was a widespread need for more information and training on such basic issues as what is dementia and how does a diagnosis of dementia relate to assessments of mental capacity in general and financial capacity in particular. Others admitted either they or their colleagues were not aware of the need for appointeeship to be taken out once mental capacity had been lost in order for someone to remain authorised to collect a pension from the post office.

Second, staff provided numerous examples of suspected financial abuse especially involving relatives, but expressed great doubt about when and how best to challenge this:

> *Where do you go next? What do you do about it? I mean the relative who will say 'well there's £4,000 came out of my mum's account into mine but she wanted me to have that money, she always said she wanted me to have that money?' – How do you then do something about that?*
>
> Quoted in Langan and Means, 1995, p44

Staff felt this dilemma to be especially acute when the missing money was small (eg keeping back some attendance allowance money) and making ripples could lead to a complete rejection of the elderly person by the relative. There was also recognition that elderly people with dementia might be exposed to financial abuse from staff coming to their homes to carry out care tasks, and that the growth of private sector home care providers made it harder to monitor this situation (Means and Langan, 1996).

Finally, staff were concerned about their own vulnerability to allegations of financial abuse. As one worker put it:

> *And that was one that did accuse me actually of taking (the money) after we'd found it and you feel very vulnerable to it you know and that was at one o' clock in the morning, when she says that we'd taken her money.*
>
> Quoted in Langan and Means, 1995, p43

The key concern of this individual and others was that it is very difficult in such circumstances to prove one's innocence.

Meeting the challenge

Social services authorities are under enormous pressure as they try to progress the community care reforms under increasingly stringent financial circumstances. However, this must not be allowed to justify a failure by local authorities to think through their policies on personal finances and elderly people with dementia. This chapter concludes with eight key questions they need to be able to answer:

What does acting on behalf of the elderly person mean?
Two issues stand out. First, is it acceptable to allow independent homes to act as appointees when their primary motivation is almost certain to be the collection of fees? Second, is it acceptable for social services authorities to place appointeeship and receivership tasks within fee collection sections of finance since this again suggests these rules are being driven by fee collection concerns rather than from the need to protect vulnerable people from financial exploitation?

What is the best balance between guidelines and procedures?
Fieldwork staff were clear they wanted more guidance and procedures relating not only to financial assessment and elderly people with dementia, but also with regard to more general money handling issues raised by those receiving care services in their own homes. Such guidance and procedures are needed badly, but equally crucial is getting the correct balance between procedures which prescribe how tasks will be carried out and guidance which offers advice in a much less prescriptive way. The danger is that senior managers will attempt to protect themselves through the production of a massive procedures manual which is impossible for field-level staff to always follow and also discouraging of creativity.

How can joint working be fostered between social services practitioners and finance/revenue staff?
Social services practitioners seem to see finance staff as only interested in money and not people, while the latter feel frustration at the failure of the former to recognise that fee income has to be collected if the 'new' community care is to work. The danger is that such negative stereotypes will feed upon themselves, creating enormous tensions to the detriment of elderly people with dementia.

Who does what? (the need to clarify roles and responsibilities)
Local authorities need to be clear about how the needs of vulnerable adults are to be met and how their wellbeing is to be monitored. This requires clarity about the roles and responsibilities of care managers/social workers, in-house service providers, independent sector providers, revenue and finance staff, and local authority inspection and monitoring staff. At the moment, there seems a danger that everybody will leave everybody else to put 'two and two together' and so carry out checks when there are reasons to be concerned.

What is mental incapacity? What is financial incapacity? What is dementia?
Social services authorities need to ensure all their staff have adequate training on the above which draws upon latest thinking (BMA/Law Society, 1995; Age Concern, 1996; Law Commission, 1995). They also need a strategy to ensure adequate training is available for the staff of independent sector service providers.

How to support elderly people with dementia in the community?
Social services authorities need to be much clearer on their policies on receivership, appointeeship and day-to-day money handling where the elderly person with dementia is living in the community. It is not adequate to concentrate just upon policy development for those in residential and nursing home care.

Do we have a coordinated response?
Social services authorities must ensure that they have a coordinated and coherent response to the full range of personal finance issues raised by elderly people with dementia such as assessment, collection of charges/fees, financial abuse and day-to-day money handling issues.

How can we value elderly people with dementia?
The coordinated response which emerges from local authorities needs to be grounded in a respect for elderly people with dementia which seeks to maximise their independence.

References

Age Concern (1996) *Resident's Money: A Guide to Good Practice in Care Homes.* London: Age Concern.

BMA/Law Society (1995) *Assessment of Mental Capacity: Guidance for Doctors and Lawyers.* London: BMA.

Centre for Policy on Ageing (1996) *A Better Home Life: A Code of Good Practice for Residential and Nursing Home Care.* London: CPA.

Langan J and Means R (1995) *Personal Finances, Elderly People with Dementia and the New Community Care*. Oxford: Anchor Trust.

Law Commission (1995) *Mental Incapacity*. London: HMSO.

Means R and Langan J (1996) Charging and quasi-markets in community care: implications for elderly people with dementia. *Social Policy and Administration* 30 (3), 244-262.

National Audit Office (1994) *Looking After the Financial Affairs of People with Mental Incapacity*. London: HMSO.

20 Home based respite care

Sue Newton

For those relatives who look after someone with dementia one of their main requests is for a break from caring. They need breaks during the day for a couple of hours at a time and longer breaks when they can go away on holiday, or visit their daughter, or attend a grandchild's christening. For people who are losing their short term memory and relying more on their long term memory the best place for them to function is in their own home. Carers do not want to cope with more disorientated and anxious behaviour from their relatives just because they have been for respite in an institution such as a hospital or a residential home. What they would often like is for someone to come and live in and look after their relative as they would. This is home based respite care.

Home based respite care (boarding-in) is an off shoot of adult placement (boarding-out). Adult placement is a very old resource in which vulnerable people, who are not related, are cared for as part of the family. It has been known of for over five hundred years but has had a recent resurgence in Britain in the last twenty years. Liverpool Personal Service Society, a voluntary social service organisation working in northwest England, has been running an adult placement scheme for respite care for older people since 1978. At first older people went to stay in scheme carers homes but as more carers requested that a scheme carer came and lived in, home based respite was developed. Scheme carers are recruited from advertisements or word of mouth from other carers. They are interviewed and assessed as to their skills and their motivation. Two references are required from someone who knows them well, as well as a reference from their doctor. They are usually older women who have a lot of experience of looking after other people either in their own personal lives or in a profession.

The scheme social worker receives referrals for respite care from district social workers, health workers or direct from the service user themselves. Having visited and assessed the needs of the informal carer and their dependent and discussed with them the various options, the scheme social worker can, if home based respite care is chosen, match the needs of the older person with the skills of the available scheme carers. Who has the experience of looking after this sort of person? Would they be able to manage this household (pets, smoking, household gadgets)? Having selected a scheme carer with the appropriate skills, the social worker arranges a pre-placement visit at which the scheme carer learns all the intricacies of daily life for the older person such as their likes and dislikes from the informal carer. Both parties would have the opportunity to find out as much as they wanted about each other. Only when everyone is satisfied does the placement go ahead. The social worker oversees the placement; monitoring and supporting where necessary.

The cost of the placement is the same as residential care. If the person is eligible the social services department fund the placement, though residential care allowance is not available when care is given in someone's own home.

When people suffering from dementia remain in their own homes, being looked after with as little change to routine as possible, the informal carer can have a break knowing that their dependent is in the best possible place. An ongoing relationship can be built up between scheme carer and older person, so that it is always the same person who comes as substitute family carer each time. Home based respite care should be an option available to all carers of people with dementia.

Further information

The National Association of Adult Placement Services,
51A Rodney Street, Liverpool, L8 0QB.

21 Elder abuse and dementia: moving forward

Lynne Phair

The abuse of older people is slowly becoming a subject that both care staff and the public are accepting as a sad reality. Many guidelines are now being developed in England following the Social Services Inspectorate guidelines developed in 1992. The purpose of these are to ensure that a multi-agency approach is taken to the management of abusive situations. However, there are few examples available of professionals working constructively with the abuser and the abused person in order to deal with the problems identified. Penhale and Kingston (1995) discuss the problem that professionals may feel inadequate to deal with abusive situations and lack strategies to do so. They also suggest that in their desire to do something to help, an inappropriate intervention may be provided.

The three case studies which follow illustrate how abuse can be dealt with positively and productively. They aim to inspire people to think about the causes of abuse and look constructively at ways of dealing with situations they may come across.

Abuse is often perceived by people, with little knowledge of the problem, to be dramatic types of physical or sexual abuse. The reality, however, is that abuse can be insidious and perhaps only come to light in a coincidental way.

The decision to intervene in situations of abuse should not be taken lightly, since adults do have a right to self-determination. For people with dementia this is no different. Professionals must decide how to maintain the balance between protection of the individual and the rights of the carer while not colluding with abusive practice or avoiding the situation.

The physical abuse of a man with dementia

A woman aged 80 years lived with her husband in a first floor flat. Mrs C was not known to the mental health or social services at all, although she had been showing signs of a dementing illness for about three years.

Mr C asked his doctor if he could have a home help to assist him with dressing his wife as he was having difficulties.

The home care manager called to arrange the services and during the interview Mr C mentioned his frustration with his wife. He would lock her in the bedroom when he could not cope any longer, and then leave the house for a couple of hours to 'calm down'. The home care manager suggested that a community psychiatric nurse (CPN) should visit in order to offer some support to Mr C. He accepted the offer a little reluctantly.

Using her skills of relationship formation and interviewing, the CPN discussed with Mr C the management of his wife when he went out. He found it difficult to express himself but acknowledged that he should not lock her up. He was at a loss about how to manage her and his frustrations. Mrs C was very affectionate towards her husband and showed no signs of any trauma.

The CPN introduced options to Mr C and asked if Mrs C could be included in the conversations. He was reluctant because of his shame, and so it was agreed that the CPN would visit and work with Mr C around a number of areas:

- education about dementia;
- management of situations that arise;
- anger management;
- support services including respite for him and Mrs C;
- supportive counselling regarding his feelings of loss, grief and shame.

The reason Mr C had gone to his GP was because he knew that resorting to physical abuse was wrong for both of them. He had never told the GP about his wife's dementia as he thought that it was just old age. This man had struggled on in the care of his wife who was unable to wash and dress herself, constantly repeated herself, yet tried to help around the house. Visits to their children used to be enjoyed but the journey had increased her confusion, so they had stopped going. Their regular trips to the pub had ceased as he felt ashamed of her. He often thought she was being awkward. Mr C wanted to care for his wife until she died. With support they both accepted the need for day care and a home help. Mr C attended the relatives' support group.

As his episodes of anger and frustration diminished, the two were able to enjoy a better quality of life together. The dementia was accepted and their lives accommodated it.

After one year Mrs C died. The CPN continued to support Mr C through his feelings of guilt of his earlier abuse for about six months after her death. Mr C slowly came to acknowledge that once he had received appropriate support, education and understanding, they had both been able to take a positive approach to a devastating situation.

This scenario illustrates how easy it is for carers who are unsupported and who have little knowledge of dementia to resort to abuse. The abuse was acknowledged and managed. Both the abuser and the abused felt supported in a way that they both wanted.

Psychological abuse of a carer

Mr A was a 74 year old retired car mechanic who had been suffering from dementia for the past four years. He had lived with his wife for forty years. Mrs A was receiving home care support as she herself had arthritis. She asked if she could see a social worker because she was finding life more difficult.

During the interview Mrs A talked of Mr A's behaviour throughout their married life. He had always been a verbally aggressive man. She expressed low self-esteem. During closer conversation she disclosed how he would torment her about her inadequacies, tell her she was useless, and accuse her of mismanaging the family finances. She used to find solace in her work as a seamstress and their two children. However, she was now less mobile. Within his progressing illness his abuse of her was increasing. She felt very depressed and suicidal at times. He would call out all night and taunt her about her disfigured hands and legs.

Mrs A felt that she needed a break, but felt powerless to take one as Mr A was dependent on her.

The social worker discussed with Mr A the need for his wife to have a break from caring. Surprisingly, Mr A realised that she was not her usual self, but had no insight into the reason why. He refused to go into any care setting as he felt that he could manage.

The social worker organised a meeting with the GP, who referred Mrs A to the CPN. The social worker then concentrated on the needs of supporting Mr A who was to remain at home whilst his wife took a break.

It was arranged that Mrs A should go to her daughters for two weeks and while she was away home helps would visit three times a day. The CPN also called in, and the GP informed his colleagues that there might be a call for assistance if Mr A deteriorated.

The respite was successful. Mrs A discussed the possibility of leaving home permanently but decided that she wanted to continue caring for her husband despite understanding how that might affect her own health. The CPN continued to work with Mrs A and to support her with counselling, social support groups and a relatives' support group; while the GP reviewed her arthritis treatment and referred her to physiotherapy. Mr A was supported by the social worker who continued to work at an emotional and practical level with him.

This package continued with intermittent respite for another eighteen months. Mrs A died and Mr A was admitted to a nursing home.

The dilemma here was the difficulty in protecting Mrs A from the psychological abuse which was causing her to experience mental health problems, while accommodating the risks to Mr A.

The case study illustrates the tightrope walked by health and social services staff when balancing the needs of both parties. It also illustrates an example of good communication and cooperation between disciplines, and risk assessment being calculated and accepted.

Abuse in an institution

An anonymous telephone call was received by the nursing home inspector in a health authority reporting that in a nursing home in her area, a patient with dementia had been force fed. Although very limited information was given, the inspector felt that all complaints should be investigated.

She visited the home the next day with a colleague and informed the matron of the complaint. Because the inspector had developed a good, open and honest relationship with the matron over the years, she was happy to work with the inspector in undertaking the investigations.

The investigation was thorough and all staff were interviewed and asked if anyone had seen anybody being fed in a rough manner. The care plans were examined to identify which patients needed help with feeding. At first the staff denied seeing anything. As the inspector gained the confidence of the staff one nurse felt able to say that she had seen a registered nurse overload a spoon of food, and silently shovel the food into the man who choked. Other staff began to come forward with reports of abusive behaviour by this nurse, including slapping patients and shouting abusive language. Slowly but surely a picture began to emerge. The nurse had used a systematic approach of physical and psychological abuse to patients in order to make them comply.

The inspector kept the matron informed and reported her findings to the police. Using Section 127 of the Mental Health Act, the police pursued the inquiry. The case came to Crown Court and the nurse pleaded guilty to five charges of ill treatment, and was jailed for fifteen months.

Caring for older people with advanced dementia is very demanding and requires many skills and considerable expertise. Staff also need appropriate support in order to help them develop their understanding. Ritualistic practice and the use of power and coercion were intrinsic in the old culture of dementia care in large institutions (Kitwood and Benson, 1995). As staff who work with people with dementia are given the opportunity to develop and adopt an individualised approach to care, their understanding of the therapeutic value of both physical and psychological care practice and the individual's right as citizens should become the standard of care everywhere.

This short chapter has illustrated, through case scenarios, how people with dementia and their carers can be supported through difficult times in a positive and productive way. The challenge is to ensure that, in the process of dealing with abuse, nobody suffers inappropriately because of the well-meant interventions of care professionals.

References

Penhale B and Kingston P (1995) Elder abuse: overview of recent and current developments. *Health and Social Care in the Community* 3(5), 311-320.

Social Services Inspectorate (1993) *No Longer Afraid: the Safeguard of Older People in Domestic Setting*. HMSO: London.

Kitwood T and Benson S (1995) *The New Culture of Dementia Care*. London: Hawker Publications.

22 Advocacy and older people with dementia

Andrew Dunning

Advocacy means making the case for someone, or a group of people, or helping them to represent their own views, usually to defend their rights or to promote their interests. The concept has special relevance to people who are disadvantaged and as a consequence are less able to speak for themselves.
Killeen, 1996

Advocacy is a process of empowerment. It has perhaps always existed within human relationships but has latterly emerged in particular forms. Brandon (1995) notes that examples in Britain include the work of John Perceval who acted as an advocate and founded the Alleged Lunatic's Friends Society in 1845. However, while advocacy for and by disabled people has begun to mushroom in more recent years, the rights and representation of older people with dementia have largely been overlooked.

The need for advocacy

The following interrelated themes have influenced interest in advocacy with this particular group.
- *Population*. Although the degree of dependency among older people is often overstated, general levels of dementia and frailty are subject to increase with age. The ageing of the population means that more of us are

likely to find ourselves in a vulnerable position. Some might not have family or friends to act as 'natural advocates', for others such relationships might be part of the problem (Wertheimer, 1993).

- *Legislation.* Advocacy has no legal status in Britain. Relevant sections of the Disabled Persons (Services, Consultation and Representation) Act 1986 which would have given individuals a statutory right to appoint a representative regarding local authority social services and other provision have not been implemented. Nevertheless, advocacy seems to be an essential element of the NHS and Community Care Act 1990 which ostensibly emphasises choice and user involvement.

- *Protection.* The role of advocacy in protecting vulnerable adults has been recognised by the Law Commission (1995) and within most adult abuse guidelines produced by health and social services authorities (Bennett and Kingston, 1993). Yet older people with dementia may also be subject to over protection and might require support in their right to take certain risks (Wynne Harley, 1991).

- *Transition.* Advocacy can be vital at particular points in time during the lives of older people with dementia. These situations include deciding on residential care; hospital discharge; decisions about hospital treatment; and closure or changes in the management of residential care homes or nursing homes (Phillipson, 1990).

- *Discrimination.* Gwilliam and Gilliard (1996) locate dementia within the social model of disability, which places ownership of disability onto society. A person has an impairment (dementia) but it is the reaction of others towards that impairment and the consequent denial of rights which is 'disabling'. As well as such disablism, older people with dementia can be confronted by ageism and a range of other types of discrimination. Advocacy attempts to challenge this position.

- *Depersonalisation.* Kitwood (1990) identifies ten 'malignant' processes and interactions which depersonalise a person with dementia: treachery, disempowerment, infantilisation, intimidation, labelling, stigmitisation, outpacing, invalidation, banishment and objectification. Advocacy is a means of ensuring that personhood is retained or reclaimed in the face of such assaults.

- *Participation.* Advocacy is about ensuring older people with dementia have the same substantive and procedural rights as other citizens. Thus, people are not just seen as users of health and social care services, but as citizens with equal rights and entitlements to a range of services and activities including housing, leisure, education, religious observance and transport facilities (Dunning, 1995).

Types of advocacy

People with dementia may need different forms of advocacy at different times, or indeed several forms over the same period. There are many types of advocacy and as each develops, distinctions can become blurred. While innovation and interconnection are vital there is a need for clarity of purpose not least so that purchasers, providers, carers and, wherever possible, the older person with dementia themselves know what is on offer. Types of advocacy may be described as follows:

Advocacy alongside/on behalf of a person/group
- Legal advocacy is perhaps the most widely known form of advocacy and is undertaken by professionally qualified lawyers on behalf of their clients.
- Professional advocacy may be undertaken by professionals such as social workers and nurses who see advocacy as part of their role. As these professionals are employed by a service providing agency conflicts of interest may arise when trying to undertake an advocacy function. There are now a growing number of workers who are paid to provide a specific independent advocacy service, such as complaints advocates and patients advocates.
- Public advocacy refers to the activities of organisations which lobby and campaign on behalf of a particular group of people, but are not necessarily controlled by those they seek to represent and often provide services themselves as part of their activities. They tend to be national bodies with local networks, such as Age Concern.
- Citizen advocacy is a one to one ongoing partnership between an independent trained volunteer citizen advocate and a person who is not in a good position to secure or exercise their rights and choices.
- Crisis advocacy shares the same principles as citizen advocacy but as its name implies is short term in nature. This tends to be one off involvement centred upon a particular task or specific situation with which a person needs support.
- Peer advocacy takes place where one person advocates for another who has experienced similar difficulties and discrimination. The Lewisham Pensioners Forum, for example, established the PALS project in which one older person advocates for another.

Advocacy by a person/group for themselves
- Self advocacy essentially means speaking up for yourself and involves a person expressing their own needs and concerns, making their own choices and decisions, and representing their own interests.

- Group or collective advocacy means a self advocacy body which offers mutual support, skill development and a common call for change. This might include a small group such as a local residents forum or large body such as the National Pensioners Convention.

Advocacy in practice: roles and models

Chapman and Marshall (1993) have called for more independent advocacy schemes for people with dementia. At present there are only a handful in existence. While, for example, there are around 170 citizen advocacy related schemes for a variety of groups in Britain, less than a dozen have a specific focus upon dementia, though some generic schemes might include older people with dementia within their remit.

On an organisational level a range of models have been developed, for example:

- Birmingham Citizen Advocacy has facilitated crisis advocacy, peer advocacy, self advocacy, group advocacy, 'professional' advocacy by project staff as well as citizen advocacy for older people with dementia and mental health problems.
- Fife Advocacy Project has similarly sought to encourage and support the development of all types of independent advocacy for the purpose of improving the life of people with dementia.
- Connect Advocacy Project in Hackney has employed a paid advocate to work with older patients on the continuing care wards of a local hospital scheduled for closure.
- Alzheimer's Disease Society Wales in Gwent offers advocacy to the person with dementia at the point of diagnosis and long term citizen advocacy beyond.

On an interpersonal level independent advocacy – paid or voluntary – involves two broad roles. First, the instrumental role within which the advocate provides practical support, undertaking tasks such as finding information, attending meetings, negotiating and securing services. Here the advocate is an information aide, troubleshooter or spokesperson. Second, the expressive role whereby the advocate provides emotional support, which may involve meeting needs through care and concern, sometimes simply 'being there'. Here the advocate can be a companion or enabler.

Advocacy in practice: challenges and opportunities

Independent advocacy currently faces a number of challenges and opportunities. Key issues relating to older people with dementia include:

'Clout'

As independent advocacy is not enshrined in law it is largely carried out at the behest of professionals. Advocacy schemes must raise awareness and negotiate protocols with purchasers and providers in order to have an impact on services. Protocols may cover matters such as maintaining independence, access to establishments, attendance at meetings, confidentiality and records.

Official guidance and debate has begun to recognise the role of independent advocacy regarding good practice in care management and assessment (SSI 1991) and older people with dementia living in the community (SSI 1996). A number of charters of rights have included access to an independent advocate within institutional settings (CPA 1996). However, a significant cultural shift in practice is still needed for advocacy to flourish.

Legislation has been implemented to create a framework for advocacy with vulnerable adults in several countries, including Australia, Canada and the USA. A package of legislation passed in Ontario in 1992 comprised a Substitute Decision Making Act, Consent to Treatment Act, an Advocacy Act and created an Advocacy Commission. Such legislation might be welcome in Britain but care would be required on a number of issues including representation on any Advocacy Commission and checks to avoid the potential misuse of power by advocates.

Capacity

On an organisational level advocacy schemes need to have 'capacity' in terms of resources to operate for the benefit of older people with dementia. Such resources include appropriate and sufficient funding (Philpot, 1993); well trained and supported advocates (Ivers, 1994); and strong community networks (Beresford and Croft, 1993). Schemes also need to beware of overestimating what they can do and avoid spreading themselves too thinly if they are to be effective (Hunter, 1995).

On an individual level an older person may lack legal capacity to take his or her own decisions. It is important to differentiate advocacy from substitute decision making. Advocacy is about finding ways to ascertain and represent a person's case and ensure that they receive their full rights and entitlements; substitute decision making involves making decisions on behalf of the person. Indeed, being an advocate in itself does not mean that an individual can give consent, sign forms or carry out legally effective acts on behalf of a partner whether that partner has capacity to take decisions or not (Dunning, 1995).

Limited legal status may be conferred on the advocate through arrangements such as Court of Protection or Guardianship where appropriate. Schemes may also meet ethical obligations and good practice considerations in being clear about whether the older person with dementia is being honestly represented on the basis of what that person is saying and 'telling it as it is', 'best interests' or 'if it were thee or me'. Otherwise they risk disempowering those they seek to represent, albeit through a kind of 'myopia of good intention' (Jack, 1995).

Communication

Goldsmith (1996) shows that the voice of people with dementia is seldom heard above the views of policy makers, professionals, care workers and carers. O'Brien (1987) suggests advocacy involves finding ways to understand, respond to and represent the person. Thus, it is vital for advocacy schemes to keep up with research in communication methods, meaning and mapping being undertaken by dementia services development centres and other specialist bodies if they are to enable the voice of older people with dementia to be heard.

Organisationally, communication must be strong between different parts of the advocacy movement and related activities. Such contacts and alliances can strengthen advocacy and widen choices for older people with dementia. Further, arrangements are required by which individual concerns can lead to systemic or structural changes, for example, between an advocacy project and a pensioners forum or local social services committee. Firm links are also needed with people from black and minority ethnic groups and others who are under represented in dementia services.

Finally, there is a need to communicate the value of advocacy by and for older people with dementia. To paraphrase the pioneering paper *Living Well into Old Age* (Kings Fund, 1986), the question is not whether advocacy can help older people with dementia, but what will their lives be like without it? Over a decade on the argument for advocacy seems all the more compelling.

References

Bennett G and Kingston P (1993) *Elder Abuse: Concepts, Theories and Interventions.* London: Chapman and Hall.

Beresford P and Croft S (1993) *Citizen Involvement: A Practical Guide for Change.* London: Macmillan.

Brandon D (1995) *Advocacy: Power to People with Disabilities.* Birmingham: Venture Press.

Centre for Policy on Ageing (1996) *A Better Home Life: A Code of Good Practice for Residential and Nursing Home Care.* London: CPA.

Chapman A and Marshall M (eds) (1993) *Dementia: New Skills for Social Workers.* London: Jessica Kingsley Publishers.

Dunning A (1995) *Citizen Advocacy with Older People: A Code of Good Practice.* London: CPA.

Goldsmith M (1996) *Hearing the Voice of People with Dementia: Opportunities and Obstacles*. London: Jessica Kingsley Publishers.

Gwilliam C and Gilliard J (1996) Dementia and the social model of disability. *Journal of Dementia Care* January/February 1996.

Hunter S (1995) Safeguarding advocacy. Unpublished paper, Department of Social Administration and Social Work, University of Edinburgh.

Ivers V (1994) *Citizen Advocacy in Action: Working with Older People*. Stoke on Trent: Beth Johnson Foundation.

Jack R (1995) *Empowerment in Community Care*. London: Chapman and Hall.

Killeen J (1996) *Advocacy and Dementia*. Edinburgh: Alzheimer Scotland Action on Dementia.

Kings Fund (1986) *Living Well into Old Age: Applying Principles of Good Practice to Services for People with Dementia*. London: Kings Fund.

Kitwood T (1990) The dialectics of dementia: with particular reference to Alzheimer's disease. *Ageing and Society* 10.

Law Commission (1995) *Mental Incapacity*. London: HMSO.

O'Brien J (1987) *Learning From Citizen Advocacy Programs*. Georgia Advocacy Office, USA.

Phillipson C (1990) Approaches to advocacy. In Bernard M and Glendenning F (eds) *Advocacy, Consumerism and the Older Person*. Stoke on Trent: Beth Johnson Foundation.

Philpot T (1993) Lip service that gags advocacy. *The Guardian*, 17 March.

Social Services Inspectorate (1991) *Care Management and Assessment: Managers' Guide*. London: HMSO.

Social Services Inspectorate (1996) *Assessing Older People with Dementia Living in the Community*. London: UK Department of Health.

Wertheimer A (1993) *Speaking Out: Citizen Advocacy with Older People*. London: CPA.

Wynne Harley D (1991) *Living Dangerously: Risk-taking, Safety and Older People*. London: CPA.

Working together

23 Bounce and balance: a team approach to risk management for people with dementia living at home

April Baragwanath

Risk is a part of life and we can no more eliminate risk for people with dementia than we can for any other member of the community. However by using a team approach to bounce ideas, perspectives and skills with family and colleagues and *balancing* the rights and risks of all those effected by a particular situation (not just the person with dementia) we can manage the risks.

Like truth, 'risk' is perceived differently by each of us: one person's risk is another person's lifestyle. This also applies to the people we live and work with who have a dementing illness. The unique life history of each person will impact on the risk management strategy developed with and for the person with dementia and their carers; there are no standard responses.

Gathering life story information about the person with dementia is crucial; it is like putting a jigsaw together. Initially the pieces do not form a picture but each additional piece of information adds to the pieces already in place. The information from the person with dementia may be limited but there are usually (but not always) other sources such as family, friends, service providers and neighbours. What can we understand about how this particular person has chosen to live their life? What gives meaning to this person's life? The risk management strategy for a retired merchant mariner or a pioneering feminist who rode through Russia on a motor cycle in the 1930s is likely to be very different from a quiet soul who has never left the village of his or her birth.

Risk management needs a proactive approach, not a reactive one dealing with perpetual crisis and emergencies. Current and potential hazards need to be identified and addressed or acknowledged as an acceptable risk in the particular situation. It has often been observed that experienced workers who are well supported develop more flexible, creative care plans for people with disabilities than inexperienced or unsupported staff. Managers need to create work environments where staff are encouraged to explore and expand the options and possibilities for people with dementia, not to unreasonably restrict their lives because of limitations of imagination and vision.

Duty of care concerns are too frequently raised by professional staff as an excuse for inadequate *individual* assessment and inflexible restrictive care plans. In some legal systems 'damages' may be seen to have occurred as a result of unreasonable restrictions being placed on the freedom and autonomy of a person with disability.

There is a widespread perception that institutional or residential care provides a risk free alternative to living at home. The presence of 24 hour staffing does not eliminate hazards. The experience of many workers in the field is that a person with dementia is more likely to injure themselves in an unfamiliar environment such as a hospital, residential respite facility or even a relative's home than their own known environment. Trying to find an unfamiliar toilet or bathroom, climbing out of a high hospital bed or over restraining cot sides coupled with the increased anxiety generated by strange people, noises and lights all increase the risk of accident or injury.

In the early 1980s Paul Brearley and others expanded on concepts borrowed from the actuarial industry for risk analysis. They looked at the key areas of the *probability* of an event occurring; the *possibility* of it occurring; the *imminence* or when an event might happen and the *gravity* of the outcome if it did occur. For example, the probability of a person dying from hypothermia in Australia is not high but is a very real risk in the UK. It is possible for a person to contact rabies in Europe but not in Australia. Could an event happen tomorrow or next year? How serious would the outcome be? Life threatening or just annoying and to whom?

Dementia does not result in a sudden global loss of abilities but a gradual and incremental loss over time. Understanding the dementing process and the difference between short term memory loss and the abilities and skills retained within the long term memory is crucial to good risk management. Careful assessment and observation will identify how the specific cognitive losses of the individual effect their ability to function *in their own particular environment* not how they function in hospital or at their daughter's house. Concerns about things which *might* happen to the person need to be evaluated in terms of possibility and probability, immanence and gravity and balanced against the actual evidence of particular concerns occurring.

A person who has been a keen fisherman all his life is likely to have water safety skills retained in his long term memory and so the regular walks to the local pier or lake may not be hazardous but may be a real risk for someone unfamiliar with water. Is there any evidence that the person behaves in an unsafe manner at the pier or lake?

In parts of rural Australia some older people still use wood stoves as their only source of cooking, heating and hot water. It would be presumptive to assume that this constitutes an unacceptable risk as many of this group have been using wood stoves all their lives and safe fire habits are deeply ingrained in their long term memory.

Relatives may relate that, 'Mum *always* leaves the gas stove on'. More specific questioning finds that this has occurred once in the last six months or maybe five times in the last week. These are very different situations requiring different responses. Perhaps a person has lost their ability to find their way home but lives in a small community where they are well known and others guide them home. Is their spatial disorientation necessarily a problem? It may be a problem in a large city but not in a small town.

Identification of the problem and who actually has the problem can be illuminating. Dressing in clothing which is climate appropriate but perhaps mismatched or eccentric may disturb others but is hardly a reason to remove someone from their home and community of many years.

One woman placed numerous tea cups on the front lawn to catch rainwater whenever it rained. The neighbours in the retirement complex found this behaviour unacceptable and requested her placement elsewhere. The behaviour was harmless and made sense in the context of her childhood in drought stricken rural Australia where water was a precious commodity. Who had the problem?

We need to identify clearly where the problem lies because it is too easy to set in motion a chain of events which result in the person with dementia bearing the consequences of someone else's problem. Interventions must be appropriately targeted. The behaviour of a person with dementia who is up at night, perhaps rummaging endlessly through clothes and cupboards, is not necessarily a problem. If they live on their own and are not disturbing others and are not lighting fires in the middle of the floor, is this a problem? However there is a problem if the person's continued care at home is dependent on a co-resident carer having adequate sleep. We need to explore ways to ensure the carer gets adequate sleep rather than automatically making the person with dementia the object of the intervention. Why sedate the person with dementia with all the concomitant problems when it is the carer who cannot sleep?

Proper nutrition and hydration are important aspects of a person's care and wellbeing but we need to be flexible in determining how this occurs. How important is it that a person eats three meals a day at certain socially determined times? Adequate intake over a 24 hour period is the key point not the times a person eats. We need to constantly challenge ourselves and the wider community to ask how important some things really are in the overall picture. Would the concern balance the losses the person might suffer if the issue is given unmerited importance? Does the gravity of the issue balance the gravity of the consequences for the person?

Occasionally workers come across elderly people who have lived isolated, reclusive lives in conditions many people would regard as substandard or at best eccentric. Changes in their behaviour as a result of a dementing illness may bring them to the attention of local services, often for the first time. Their chosen lifestyle may not sit comfortably with mainstream society but it is paternalistic and often absurd to argue that such an environment constitutes a risk or health hazard when the person is 85 years old, in excellent physical health and has lived this way for the last fifty years.

A very contentious issue relates to a person with dementia who lives alone and is inclined to wander, especially at night. Is it acceptable practice to lock the doors knowing the person would be unable to unlock them in an emergency? Balancing the pros and cons of the individual situation are critical. There is an acknowledged risk of the person being trapped in the house in the event of a fire. Minimising the risk of fire would be part of the care plan but it cannot be eliminated. The risk of the person wandering from home at night, often inadequately dressed and vulnerable to traffic accidents, exposure or assault, may be a high probability event if the doors are not secured. Does the low probability of fire justify removing someone from a loved home and garden to a new and unfamiliar environment when this is contrary to the known wishes of the person with dementia? Where does the balance lie for this particular person?

This is a very real dilemma for family and professional workers where balancing the risk probabilities against the quality of life issues for the person needs the input of several people brainstorming ideas and views. The team includes the person with dementia, their family and carers as well as professional staff. These are big issues and such decisions are best shared. Families and work places need to develop a culture that encourages open communication and support as a sign of strength and professional development. None of us have all the answers and it is an opportunity to grow and develop, to learn from our clients, their families and carers as well as our colleagues.

Sadly, but inevitably, there will be instances where there is a tragic outcome for a client or family member. It is important that family and workers involved are supported by colleagues and supervisors to accept that despite the best care planning and risk management strategies when we are working with people we cannot eliminate risk from anybody's life, including our own.

Supporting people with dementia to live the closing chapters of their lives safely and in a way which affirms their dignity and individuality and is congruent with the way they have chosen to lead their lives in the past is a challenge for both family carers and workers.

One sunny Sunday morning one of our clients, a woman in her eighties with moderate dementia who lived alone, was observed by neighbours walking round her garden talking to her flowers.
An hour later she was found by her friend who called to take her to church lying on her bed. She had died as she wished, with her home and garden around her.

Bouncing ideas and dilemmas with trusted colleagues and friends to achieve a balance between the rights and risks, the important and the not so important, for a person with dementia is good practice – in life as well as in work.

24 Joint working: the impossible dream?

Valerie Good

What kind of care do people with dementia need and who should provide it?

It is obvious to most carers of people with dementia that they and the person they care for have a unique combination of needs that change over time, sometimes subtly, sometimes dramatically. The services they are likely to need will include elements of the following:
- financial and welfare rights advice;
- help with domestic tasks;
- the diagnosis and treatment of physical illnesses;
- information about the illness and its effects;
- assistance with personal care tasks;
- advice about risk management;
- respite care – either residential or day respite;
- longstay care;
- counselling and support.

The majority of the population have only a passing understanding of the complexities of 'welfare' organisations, with a hazy appreciation of who provides what. Usually the first time you think about how health and social care is provided is when you or a family member are in some sort of crisis.

Imagine that you are a carer who is suddenly faced with a diagnosis of dementia in a family member, you may think the hardest thing will be to decide what service will help you most. You probably will not comprehend at first that these services are provided by a whole range of organisations but as time goes on you will come to realise that the provision of the first two items on the list were traditionally the responsibility of social services departments and that prior to the National Health Services and Community Care Act (1990) these services would have been provided directly by their staff. The need for a proportion of community care monies to be spent in the 'independent' sector has encouraged many social services departments to contract out these services to a number of independent providers. The third service on the list is the sole province of health but the remaining services on the list form a 'grey area' and could be provided by either agency. As a carer you will discover by talking to others in similar situations that the route of referral and the traditions of the locality will dictate the style, quality, quantity, cost and the supplier of the services provided. You will also hear, in the worse scenarios, of poor working relationships between health and social care professionals, rivalry between organisations and a complex morass of uncoordinated paperwork. This kind of piecemeal approach to the provision of care for people with dementia is neither acceptable, effective nor efficient.

The majority of carers of people with dementia are neither greedy nor unrealistic, all they want are services that are timely, tailored to their specific needs and provided in an appropriate manner. They do not want to spend their time working out which agency to badger, or deciding which professional supplies can be provided by which service. Carers rarely have much sympathy for the rationale behind the current division of social care services and health care. Instead of a 'seamless care package' they hear constant arguments over *who* should provide *what* and whether the various elements of services are *free* or *charged for*. Examples of these situations abound:

> *Mrs Boyd, a woman with dementia, has just been discharged from a day hospital where she had a full and thorough multidisciplinary assessment. She now needs to attend day care to give her carer a much needed break. She is visited by a social services care manager who may be unfamiliar with the problems that can be associated with dementia. The care manager has to complete a lengthy assessment before the care can be provided. The previous assessment is disregarded.*

Mrs O'Malley has dementia and is living alone at home. She needs close supervision and assistance with her medication. Home helps visit several times a day and a community psychiatric nurse (CPN) calls weekly; they sometimes meet on the doorstep, at other times they may not see each other for months. They keep separate records and neither is sure who is reordering the medicines. How does the GP get accurate information about the effectiveness of the medication?

Mr Stewart has dementia and rarely sleeps through the night. His worn out carer needs frequent respite. Who decides whether 'free' hospital respite, or 'means tested' social respite is provided.

If high quality dementia care requires a coordinated approach idea why doesn't it happen more often?

Nearly every example of good practice in collaborative working between health and social services can be traced back to the initiative of a small number of key local people. Collaboration has rarely occurred as a result either of legislation or national policy and the substantial cultural differences of the two agencies present substantial barriers to all but the bravest.

In spite of this difficulty a number of joint initiatives were established in the late 1980s that demonstrated that a 'seamless service' and a 'one door' point of access to services for older people with mental health problems were both popular with users and capable of providing innovative, high quality and cost effective services. Most of these services were successful because they ignored traditional professional boundaries and responded to individual need by deploying staff appropriately regardless of the agency that employed them.

Many of us who work with people with dementia saw these schemes as the model for future services. We looked forward in anticipation to the implementation of the National Health Service and Community Care Act naively thinking that the objectives of this new legislation would lead to the possibility of an integrated approach to dementia care. It might have done except for four substantial problems:

- the Act introduced 'the mixed economy', 'care management' and 'holistic assessment' but did nothing to ensure that health and social service departments would have to work closer together. The two agencies were required to agree on a number of issues including 'discharge from hospital' protocols but there were no mechanisms described in the legislation that would lead the agencies to achieve the degree of understanding, trust and mutual respect necessary for collaborative working;

- the Act encouraged social services departments to purchase a large proportion of their services. The need for health trusts to generate income has caused many of them to develop services 'for sale' and has given rise to some situations where health trusts are in direct competition for 'social care' work against social service department in-house providers;
- since the Act was implemented both health authorities and social services departments have been facing constant budgetary pressure. Clearly when bureaucracies face lean times one of their first actions will be to reinforce and clarify the boundaries of their responsibility in the belief that an effective way of saving money is to be explicit about what you do *and what you do not do*. In some areas dementia care has been redefined as a 'social issue', leaving health services to concentrate their efforts on older people with functional illnesses;
- the internal market in health care has forced health trusts to compete for contracts specified by health authorities. These authorities are now the customer who must be satisfied; the patient is merely the raw material to be processed. Contracts are increasingly explicit, thus minimising the opportunity to exploit the 'grey areas' of care. A CPN may have been very willing to sit with domiciliary care colleagues and help them devise an effective way of maintaining an older person with dementia at home. Now the CPN may have problems in accounting for this non-client contact time.

What ever happened to joint commissioning?

The National Health Service and Community Care Act did propose that services should be jointly commissioned. This approach would have been eminently suited to dementia services. Unfortunately, although much has been written about the merits of this approach, there has been little action. The rhetoric tended to underestimate the difficulty of getting two very different organisations to work together.

In reality there seems to be a wide diversity of opinion about what 'joint commissioning' really means, in particular there is little clarity or universal acceptance about the processes required. Central to any successful joint commissioning is the notion of a joint budget. This may be a simple and obvious concept to most carers and practitioners but it appears to be a terrifying prospect to most finance officers who seem to have an increasing influence in the market driven approach. Their anxiety is compounded by talk of a tidal wave of older people, many with dementia, waiting just around the corner with the potential to overwhelm the budgets of any caring agency. What is needed is a change of mindset so that joint working and joint commissioning is seen as a cost effective solution to a range of problems rather than an unaffordable and high risk luxury. This approach relies on putting the needs of individual people with dementia and their carers at the very centre of the planning process.

The steps to success

In the light of this disarray it is easy to do nothing and await the inevitable day when (hopefully) health and social care agencies are merged. In spite of organisational problems, I would argue that there are things that can be done now that will improve the situation of people with dementia. The suggestions include actions appropriate for all levels of staff:

- begin to develop a local strategy for dementia services – start with getting agreement on a statement of principles and values;
- talk about the grey areas with colleagues from both agencies – try to establish who is best placed to do what. Are staff in both agencies clear about each others priorities, criteria and skills;
- establish close working relationships with operational staff in your locality. Get members of staff to shadow each other in order to gain more insight into each other's organisation and culture;
- audit the care being provided to a group of service users, how many people have elements of health and social care? Can the services be reconfigured to make them more appropriate. For example if someone needs assistance to go to bed at 10.30pm and the home help service stops at 10.00pm can the community nursing service provide the service if home helps take on an additional getting up call?
- develop a group that looks at practice issues – staff from different organisations are often surprised how many 'problems' they have in common. Start a multidisciplinary quality circle;
- establish a Dementia Care Mapping team with members drawn from both agencies. Offer to audit sites operated by both organisations;
- share training opportunities across professional boundaries;
- ensure that staff have time and encouragement to develop and maintain networks;
- talk regularly to carers and involve them in your plans for service development;
- if relationships between the agencies is really difficult try to get groups such as the Alzheimer's Disease Society and Age Concern to act as mediators;
- a cooperative culture may be helped to develop and flourish if a way is found to celebrate and disseminate information about individual examples of successful collaborative care provision.

Everybody offering a service to people with dementia, no matter what their position in the organisation, can make a difference and can affect the prospect of joint working for good or ill.

The vast majority of staff in both social services departments and in health authorities and trusts are highly motivated and desperately wish to provide a good service. There are substantial frustrations attached to working with such a challenging illness particularly when resources are tight; staff groups need to ensure that they do not heap unwarranted blame or criticism onto other agencies and other staff groups. The task of developing a seamless service may be neither simple nor quick but the prize of knowing that you are providing the best possible service within your resources is well worth the effort.

25 Which hat should we wear today? Recruiting and developing the ideal workforce for dementia care

Gill Herbert

Who do we need for what?

Caring for people with dementia and supporting relatives or friends who care for them at home are now integral parts of any health or social service for older people. In designing such services, we have increasingly focused on the most appropriate workforce skill mix but we tend to make this judgement on the basis of peoples' qualifications and professional background rather than on their interests and general abilities.

We have begun to question the use of highly paid qualified staff for the bulk of care work, primarily on the ground of cost, and in so doing we have enraged those committed professionals who not only value the knowledge and skill base that their training has given them but question the assumption that less well-trained staff can offer acceptable standards of care. We have however learned also to appreciate and value the unqualified or informal care worker who, with a little training and support, is often the one person able to understand, respond to and communicate with the person with whom they spend so much of their time.

The calls in the press in recent months for the recognition of professional skills in longstay care and community care services raise many questions about what a generic care worker can and should be allowed to do; these at times reflect some of the unions' obsessions with job demarcations during the industrial disputes of the 1960s.

Those of us observing a wide range of dementia care in the last decade are acutely aware that the rigid delineation of professional skills is often detrimental to the way in which care staff (used in its generic term to cover all professionally qualified and unqualified staff) respond to people with dementia in creating a good living environment where they feel comfortable and cared for. What is important is the combination of attitudes with which the person with dementia is faced in the course of their journey through the day, and the way in which those around them work together to smooth the difficulties which arise.

Challenging behaviour, aggression and other antisocial activity exhibited by people with dementia are often a reflection of the mismatch of expectations placed upon them and their inability to influence or control things in any other way. By creating an environment in which the expectations are clear, consistent, applied by all carers and care workers, and reasonable in terms of what the individual can and cannot do, carers and care workers can significantly improve individuals behaviour and responsiveness. This can often be done as well by relatives, friends and volunteers as by highly qualified professionals. It is the attitude and approach they take to the care they provide which primarily governs the wellbeing of the person they care for as much as their technical or professional knowledge.

Learning from carers

We can learn a lot from listening to the families and carers of people with dementia about the ways in which they have discovered what is important as the people they care for change. It is often only painstaking trial and error alongside frequent observation which will reveal the way in which to divert current anxieties with responses which reassure and soothe. We can and must apply this learning to workforce training and development. Informal carers are not selected for their skills; and although most are able to cope with some aspects of caring, many discover areas where they need help to develop and learn how to approach things differently if they are to manage the care task well. In understanding how best to support them in their caring, we can learn too how best to provide professional services, whether in specialist care settings or generic services.

Currently, many of our staff are no more dementia care specialists than their neighbours who care for their relatives and friends at home. Our highly qualified nurses, psychologists, psychiatrists, social workers and managers do not usually have the patience or time to really get to know the detailed daily experiences and responses of the people who need care. What they can do is apply their theoretical expertise, their accumulated experience and knowledge, their managerial and organisational skills, and their creativity and wisdom to create environments in which care workers and cared for can learn to live with each other more harmoniously and with better understanding.

However, they can only do this if the care workers offering daily care and support can observe, feed back information and respond to suggestions of alternative approaches from the professionals supporting them. This can only happen where there is trust in the relationship and the views of the carers and care workers are treated with respect by the professionals; recognising indeed that it is often their views which contribute to learning and development of new ideas. This applies as much to care workers in a residential home, to auxiliary staff in hospital wards, to home care workers and to volunteers running day centres as it does to relatives and friends who offer the bulk of home based care. So how can we decide the combination of skills that are needed in the people who care and the people that support the carers and care workers?

In planning the ideal workforce for any service, whether it be longstay care in a residential or nursing home environment, a domiciliary care service, a day centre or a service to support informal carers in their task (be that a team of community nurses or an information service), it may be helpful to consider what is needed in terms of attitudes as well as skills, and what individuals are needed in a team to achieve the right balance.

Skills needed for dementia care

A few ideas follow on what skills count in the ideal workforce providing a service which includes care workers who can respond well to people with dementia. I am sure there are many which could be added by carers and professionals:

- *observational skills* – ability to notice if someone is content, discontent, has changed in any particular way, or is reacting differently;
- *practical care skills* – understanding the way in which personal care tasks are felt by those unable to tell you; knowing what is needed and what is preferred;
- *interpretive skills* – recognising when a response could be a reaction to pain; connecting a current behaviour to a past event or routine; picking up meaning in apparent gibberish;
- *communication skills* – being able to reassure someone unable to understand what you are saying; encouraging cooperation rather than imposing care; listening to what is being communicated, even if unable to understand what is being said;
- *planning and organisational skills* – thinking through what aspects of the environment or activity programmes may become distressing for an

elderly person with dementia; connecting the person to the routines and activities of daily living not imposing them; providing a varied but comfortable combination of routines and rituals with stimulating but not threatening innovations;

- *interpersonal and group work skills* – understanding the effects people have on each other; being able to help people help each other;
- *design and furnishing skills* – recognising the way in which particular physical features of the building may affect the wellbeing of the person with dementia, for example positioning of mirrors, ease of access to the lavatory, individualised environments which reflect preferences, lighting, colours and textures;
- *management skills* – supporting and encouraging others to do what they do better and understanding the help they need to do it; ensuring that people and facilities are employed to best effect and carers and care workers have everything they need to care well.

Attitudes needed for dementia care

But none of these skills are any use if those in day-to-day contact with people with dementia – the carers and care workers and others offering this range of professional skills and support – do not have the appropriate attitudes. The most successful informal caring partnerships are evident when carers have developed the following attitudes:

- an ability to value the person they care for regardless of their behaviour, their ability to communicate by normal means or their social skills;
- an interest in improving the quality of life of the person they care for no matter how difficult the challenges may be;
- a willingness to try and try again – good dementia care is all about inform-ed trial and error and having the confidence to accept that a totally different approach may be needed;
- a tolerance of repetitive, apparently meaningless, irritating and sometimes hurtful approaches from the person cared for together with an under-standing that it is not intentional but is founded in misinterpretation or misunderstanding of their experience of their world;
- an understanding of when, as a carer, they have had enough and need to regenerate by letting someone else take over caring for a while.

We need to ensure that the ability to develop these attitudes in the workforce is regarded as an essential skill ingredient in any team, and encourage the workers and carers in developing their own approaches to achieve these attitudes.

Putting it together – developing the team

While we continue to think of recruitment and workforce planning only in terms of the training and qualifications of the individuals we need to employ, we may miss a fundamental aspect of delivering good dementia care. It is the collective impact of the team which manages, advises and supervises the workforce in day-to-day contact with the person with dementia which determines the experience of the person cared for. No one member of the team will be able to acquire all the skills and attitudes listed above, or support others in acquiring them, but together they need to be able to offer whatever the workforce of care workers need. In recruiting new people, achieving the overall balance in both skills and attitudes should be the aim. In developing individuals, the aim should be to widen their range of abilities and approaches in responding to others. It is also particularly important to ensure that someone takes full responsibility for the collective impact of the team on the individuals they care for.

What we need and what we should be paying for are managers and professionals with the skills to motivate, develop and support carers and care workers into providing this level and approach to day-to-day care. Their teams will also be supported by people with technical skills to medically assess, diagnose and treat conditions which exacerbate the symptoms and intellectual devastation caused by dementing illness; people with specialist expertise to advise and counsel; and all the skills that the therapeutic and healthcare professionals can offer alongside the social development skills listed above. They do not all need to be available at all times.

It is those who manage and coordinate the support of the carers and care workers in this way that are the foundation on which community care and long-term care provision need to be built in order to ensure that we have services able to care for people with dementia as human beings with increasing disabilities, who have individual needs and preferences and who respond differently and often unpredictably to their world and those in contact with them. The challenge is to discover how best to recruit, develop and support the teams that can achieve this.

26 Demolishing the barriers: community dementia team development in Coventry

David Sheard

People with dementia and their carers need services which make sense. Emphasis in the 1990s is on the development of 'seamless' services. Merging best practice in health and social services is not easy and begins with the development of a joint strategy involving all interested groups. Coventry has spent the last twelve years forging a 'single management model' of its budgets, staffing and resources to achieve an integrated community dementia service. This has challenged traditional health and social services methods of working but is a model that makes sense.

When people with dementia or their carers are asked what is their experience of seeking help from health and social services too often their reply will be:

- 'I did not know where to go to get help';
- 'So many people have come knocking at my door asking the same questions';
- 'I have had a large number of different assessments all with their own forms';
- 'I have so many different telephone numbers to get hold of different professionals';
- 'I have to go to different offices to get help from health and social services';
- 'I am tired of repeating the same information to hospital staff and to people who visit me';
- 'I did not feel confident my individual, racial, cultural or religious needs were being addressed';
- 'I found my relative being unnecessarily transferred from one hospital to another which increased their confusion'.

Recognising these difficulties, a variety of different 'models' of community dementia teams have developed across the country (Abendorff et al, 1994). These 'teams' have ranged from loose networks of health and social services staff to multidisciplinary teams with or without a manager. With the advantages of coterminosity Coventry Social Services Department and Coventry Healthcare National Health Service Trust have gone one step further. In addition to developing three community mental health teams for older people comprising forty staff, they have merged the management of these teams with all old age psychiatry inpatient and day hospital services through a single management approach.

This has meant positively grasping the nettle of different organisational cultures and professional working practices to merge the best of the past alongside meeting the challenges of true integration of all health and social services resources. Across the country mental health services have faced fresh demands posed by implementation of the care programme approach and community care legislation. With the emergence of general practitioner fundholding, Coventry has responded by ensuring these developments are 'bolted on' to its model of provision enhancing the single service approach rather than risking fragmentation of a multidisciplinary model.

Getting started

Coventry Social Services Department and Coventry Health Authority established their first Community Support Team in 1984 for older people with an organic or functional mental health problem. In Coventry the total number of people aged over 65 with estimated prevalence of dementia was approximately 3,500. The team comprised a social worker, occupational therapist, psychologist, community psychiatric nurse, administrative officer and a home care organiser with associated care staff. Overseen by a multi-agency group the team of highly committed professionals quickly developed the service's reputation gaining a *Community Care* journal award in 1987. At this stage the team was neither consultant-led, though it had consultant psychiatrist input, nor had a team manager, but it had a rotating team coordinator from within its members. The team was housed in an annexe building on the site of a day centre and nursing home for people with dementia. Its catchment area was city-wide. Characterised by innovation and significant direct support to people with dementia and people with a functional mental health problem, its development was still hampered by lack of strategic direction, lack of common administrative and record systems and, to a degree, maintenance of professional barriers through separate management accountability and budgets.

Strategic development

By 1992 the Community Support Team comprised four community mental health nurses, two social workers, one occupational therapist, one psychologist and one administrative officer. The attached specialist home care services had been devolved into the Social Services Department District Office Home Care

Service. It is from this point that the development of the single management model can be tracked.

Single Management Model

1992   Allocation of Mental Illness Specific Grant to enable:
- First appointment of Team Manager
- Commissioning of second Team
- Teams renamed to Community Mental Health Teams (Older People)
- Team Manager member of Old Age Psychiatry Directorate Management Team and Social Services Department District Management Team
- Team Manager accountable to Social Services Department Assistant
- Director and Chief Executive Community and Mental Health Unit

1993   Allocation of Mental Health Development Programme monies to increase size of the two teams

1994   Team Manager role becomes General Manager – Old Age Psychiatry within the fourth wave National Health Service Trust (managing the two teams, inpatient and day hospital services – accountable to Director of Operations within the Trust and with a reporting line to Assistant Director Social Services Department

1995   Team Managers appointed to each of the two Community Mental Health Teams (Older People) accountable to the General Manager, Old Age Psychiatry
- Coventry Health monies allocated to commission third Team
- Third Team Manager appointed
- Moves for the three Community Mental Health Teams (Older People) workers to be linked to General Practitioners

Management model – key features

A number of key features were required to achieve this single management model and these were developed between 1992 and 1995:
- *joint commissioning* – with health and social services jointly purchasing development of the teams and services within old age psychiatry;
- *establishment of a single contract* – for the three teams developed within the old age psychiatry service to hold a contract on activity as part of the National Health Service Trust's annual cycle of business planning and contracting;

- *multidisciplinary management* – all team manager posts were open for any discipline to apply;
- *team acceptance* – that all team staff would be managed by the one manager regardless of background;
- *links with professional head* – for team manager and individual staff to receive support;
- *dual reporting structure* – for the team manager to report both to social services department and the trust and have membership of both agencies management teams;
- *partnership between General Manager and Clinical Coordinator* – that the medical and bio/social models of old age psychiatry are linked and represented in a partnership of these two posts within the trust heading up the old age psychiatry management team;
- *transfer of budgets* – for the team manager to hold all staffing budgets and follow the financial regulations and personnel requirements of both agencies;
- *integration with Mental Health Unit* – for the three teams to follow the service user in/out of the inpatient/day hospital service taking responsibility with staff in these settings for the implementation of Care Programme Approach and its integration with Assessment and Care Management;
- *common assessment model* – all team members/disciplines developed and used the same assessment tool/documentation;
- *approved social worker* service – managed and provided from within the three teams enabling swift and knowledgeable assessment;
- *multidisciplinary care management* – for the social services department to accept all team members/disciplines to act as care managers directly purchasing care on behalf of the social services department;
- *integrated IT systems* – for all team staff to design, develop and use one information technology system across all disciplines and both agencies thus meeting both agencies' information requirements: this involved practitioner input into computer terminals on a new arm of Coventry Social Services Department's information technology system;
- *carer/service user consultation exercises* – to ensure that the service developments are needs-responsive.

These features have not evolved in one stroke and require significant cooperation at practitioner level and senior management levels to come together into a working model. Most importantly they required both the healthcare trust and the social services department to adapt their management and central support structures, ie personnel, finance, administration and IT to enable the teams to function. Thus removing the more traditional boundaries within these structures which could have impeded their progress. It is interesting to note that a significant proportion of the integrated approach was service-driven. It would be difficult to assess whether the subsequent emergence of joint commissioning would have been able to commission such a service.

The gains for dementia care

So has this model addressed the experiences and concerns of people with dementia and their carers? Like most other community dementia services Coventry's approach has gone largely undocumented and has not been evaluated. Independent visits by bodies such as the Mental Health Act Commission and the Health Advisory Service have spoken highly of the service. The existence of innovation and much anecdotal evidence from service users and carers – including satisfaction surveys and carer interviews – supports the development of these teams.

What can service users and carers expect?

The service encourages the direct contact of the person with dementia and the carer through an open referral system. A keyworker is allocated as their one point of reference and support, the keyworker's role being to coordinate any assessment, specialist advice or practical help/services they require. This involves only contacting one place – the team base. Access is automatically available to an emergency service/advice line run across the three teams. If they are placed on a waiting list a published priority system with clear time standards exists which indicates when they should receive help. The emphasis will be on the assessment and diagnosis occurring in the community with inpatient admission only for the most complex diagnoses. The team staff all contribute to one case file and record system.

Developing new services

With the foundations in place to provide an integrated 'seamless' service new developments in services have also occurred. The teams have successfully recruited Asian and African Caribbean staff to develop a strategy for mental health service provision for black elders and their carers/communities. An outreach project within the teams into the Acute Hospital Trust to provide assessment and prevent unnecessary hospital transfers has run for two years. Continuing investment by both health and social services department purchasers has allowed refurbishment of the inpatient and day hospital service alongside the development of the Snoezelen approach and Dementia Care Mapping. The use of patients'councils and an advocacy service has been one feature of a partnership with the local branch of the Alzheimer's Disease Society. There is a wide range of day care services provided through a variety of statutory and independent sector providers.

Lessons learned and future challenges

A high profile community based mental health service for older people will present its challenges. The service is estimated in any one year to work with approximately 1,200 people of whom 50 per cent will have an organic illness, the remaining 50 per cent a functional mental health problem.

- teams faced with these competing needs cannot concentrate solely on dementia care and there can be dangers that the specific needs of people with dementia are lost in wider mental health issues;
- concentration on high quality 'seamless' assessment and care planning can be at the cost of long-term continuity of support necessary for those with a degenerative illness. The introduction of community care measures into the teams created a split in the teams between 'assessors' undertaking comprehensive assessments and 'providers' of therapeutic treatment and support. With hindsight this emphasised an over-concentration on assessment to the detriment of therapeutic support and created a meaningless split in team roles to people with dementia and their carers;
- staff in the teams can feel overwhelmed at meeting the community care requirements of social services departments alongside national health service trust contract requirements. Streamlining of these different sets of demands is required;
- not all staff are suited to these forms of multidisciplinary working preferring to retain their distinct professional skills rather than risk becoming a generic mental health worker;
- multidisciplinary teams in secondary settings appear not to have been as successful as required in working more closely with general practitioners and primary care teams. This has brought with it dangers of fragmentation as general practitioners consider purchasing a more traditional community psychiatric nurse model for dementia care;
- creative tensions can arise between the demands of accountability of the general manager to two organisations with the need for the consultant clinical coordinator of the service to set the clinical direction within the Trust.

A wide range of new issues confronts staff once barriers are demolished:

- will social services departments, in creating all disciplines as care managers, also transfer care management budget responsibility to the general manager, to the Trust or retain that portion of management?
- will the social services department have an equal part in joint agency

service contract negotiations held between the Trust and the health purchasers?

- will the community teams be better sited in newly emerging community mental health resource centres for all age groups and be more locality managed?

These remain structural issues to be resolved. Demolishing any barriers brings with it freedom and also uncertainty. This is the case in health and social care. Coventry has bravely begun demolishing these barriers to work towards its dementia care services making sense.

References

Abendorff/Challis and Netten (1994). Staff activity patterns in a community mental health team for older people. *International Journal of Geriatric Psychiatry* 9, 897-906.

Barber/Dormer and Prasadu (1996) Developing flexible, responsive teamwork. *Journal of Dementia Care* 4(1), 26-27.

Editorial Comment (1995). Can multidisciplinary teams carry out competent and safe psychogeriatric assessments in the community. *International Journal of Geriatric Psychiatry* 10, 173-177.

Junaid/Bruce (1994). Providing a community psychogeriatric service: models of community psychiatric nursing provision in a single health district. *International Journal of Geriatric Psychiatry* 9, 715-720.

Wilcox/Jones and Alldrick (1995). Identifying the support needs of people with dementia and older people with mental illness on a Joint Community Team: A preliminary report. *Journal of Mental Health* 157-163.

27 Dementia care management: healing the split

Phyllis J Sturges

Introduction

It is well known that maintaining those with dementia in the community is one of the most complex operations and certainly the most expensive in all of community care (Challis and Davies, 1986). As Gilhooly (1989) has commented, 'elderly dementia sufferers are significantly different than other groups'. Therefore, interventions to assist them at home need to be specialised as well. For carers this is the most difficult kind of care giving. Like chronic mental illness, this is a family disease and can take a heavy toll on everyone involved. Interventions for carers also need a specialised approach.

All developed countries are struggling with long term care and with the best ways to work with both people with dementia and their carers. The costs, both in the community and in institutions are enormous. The USA, for example, has been estimated to spend eighty billion dollars per year on dementia (US Congress, 1987). With greater numbers of older people in the future, these kinds of costs cannot be sustained. As the search for a cure continues, there is still the task of providing assistance for those already afflicted. The fact that most carers are women, often working outside the home or in poor health themselves, makes this an important gender issue as well.

Dysfunctional community care

In order to be effective, community based dementia care must provide a seamless service. Because it is a mental disorder, effective assessment and intervention requires the integration of health, social services and housing. Early intervention, education, home services, social support and respite are needed. Sadly, the great problem of community care, aside from being seriously under resourced, is the poor interface between health and social services. A separate mental health agency has been proposed in order to deal with this problem. Whether one agrees with this idea or not, it's not surprising that it has been suggested. The lack of coordination for those having mental disorders, including dementia, has become desperate.

What currently exists are a host of fragmented community services. Outside of health facilities, those with dementia and their carers may or may not receive the kind of help they need including an adequate diagnosis. Government Guidance on community care did not suggest ways to do outreach to vulnerable and isolated individuals and families nor did it encourage targeting for vulnerable groups. In my judgment, this was a serious error with negative consequences for people with dementia and their carers.

Community based geriatric mental health teams work with those with dementia but they are part of a general case load. As such, they may sink to the bottom in terms of priority. Care managers working in social work departments see those with dementia, but again these cases are part of a general case load. Care managers often do not work on old age mental health teams either, therefore purchasing power is split off from health care.

Psycho-geriatricians are usually working inside institutional facilities and too few are doing community based work. Therefore they are less available as a resource to field workers. GPs see the majority of those with dementia, as well as their carers, but vary considerably in their expertise in working with this group. Some refer on for specialised diagnosis and treatment, but many do not. More effort is needed in working with GPs as they are the major referral source, but this is rarely done in any systematic way.

Professionals in acute care and longstay hospitals who are working in the discharge or resettling of dementia patients usually do not have a specialised team to which to refer individuals and families. As a result, many individuals are ending up in nursing homes which often provide poorer care than they received in the psycho-geriatric wards they left. Carers fare little better. Much lip service was given to their needs in the community care policy documents and legislation, but the reality is that services for them are diffuse and underfunded. Wistow (1995) has argued that carers may be worse off now than before because of the closure of longstay hospital beds and new charging policies for home and institutional care.

Dementia care management teams

All is not gloom and doom, however, because of the promising innovation of dementia care management teams. My research in the past five years (Sturges, 1994, 1996) studied the structural and practice issues of these teams. The research has convinced me that this kind of targeted care management is required for effective community care in dementia. There are a variety of models of dementia care management, but I will describe here the model which appears to be the most functional. Not only does this model provide the kinds of coordinated help which those people with dementia and their carers need, it also has the potential to heal the split between health and social services in this area.

The teams do this through their structure, which represents a pooling of funds and personnel from both sectors. The best teams that I have seen have a specialised staff: a psychiatric nurse trained in dementia care, a qualified social worker with experience with elderly people, support staff, and back up from a psycho-geriatrician. The teams also have a corps of home care workers (Rees and Sennett, 1992; Gordon Dementia Team, 1995). These workers have a broad and flexible remit. They do personal care as well as house work as needed, and they also provide respite and social support to carers. These are the services which research has showed are most needed by people with dementia and their carers (Levin et al, 1989; Bass et al, 1996).

Referrals are received from anyone in the community and are screened. Assessments are done jointly by both the nurse and the social worker. A case load of around forty is held jointly by the team and the nurse and social worker trade off being the care manager depending on whether the problem is predominantly health related or more psycho-social. The nurse and social worker are the team leaders; there appears to be little reason for the leader to be a physician.

The teams find that they need to identify clients in the early stages of the disease. The experience of the EPIC project as reported by Bland (1996) showed that GPs often did not refer until the disease was well advanced and then little could be done. In a thoughtful discussion of user choice with people with dementia, Winner (1996) describes why early contact is also important in order to ascertain user's needs and desires. Early identification means education and support can be provided which can forestall more serious problems later on. Over time the number and intensity of services can be increased as the disease progresses. The pace is that of the individual and of the carer. Care packages might include home care, perhaps a support group, day services if desired, appliances if needed, and respite of various kinds. My research on care management in the US has indicated that well trained and supervised volunteers can also be used to assist in monitoring, provide support to users and carers and provide respite (Sturges, 1985, 1986).

The care workers provide the home services and some of the respite. In the Welsh team there was a very low rate of illness and turnover among the home care workers because they saw themselves as part of the team and had long term relationships with families. They liked the fact that their roles were flexible and changed as the needs of clients changed. Such evidence should be considered when research looks at cost effectiveness, since turnover among home care workers is a serious and expensive problem in long term care.

Monitoring is crucial to this model, although care management in Britain has tended to misunderstand its importance. Regular face to face and telephone contacts, and weekly staffings, not just periodic reviews, are required. This is an intensive clinical model of care management which is required in community work with those with dementia. It is a distinct contrast to the administrative style which is more prevalent in local authority social work departments today (Challis et al, 1990; Sturges, forthcoming).

In this clinical model counselling is often needed. Carers are known to be high users of mental health services and family differences over care may sometimes require family work. The decision to institutionalise is also an important one. There is no good reason to refer this kind of work out unless long term treatment or medication is required. Nor is it especially functional to designate one member of the team to do it. Both nurse and social worker should be trained and expected to provide counselling.

A purchaser/provider split makes no sense in a consolidated model of care such as this. Dementia care management must both purchase and provide services, as GPs also do. Any attempts to do this kind of work and to separate functions will not be effective and should not be attempted. Replications of the team model without such provider services as home care and counselling should also be avoided.

What seems astonishing is that planners and managers do not seem to recognise what an important innovation dementia care management is. It is unique to Britain insofar as I have been able to ascertain, but is a model which every country involved in community based long term care could try out. Its use in Britain is uncertain, despite such successful projects as the Coventry team which is described by David Sheard in this volume. Only Wales seems to have embraced the concept more comprehensively.

There is debate about whether resources should be spent on high quality institutional care or on community based care (Bland, 1996). The real issue is that there needs to be choice and that is what a well functioning dementia care management team can provide. Premature institutionalisation because of a lack of home services, poorly coordinated care, or caregivers without support can be prevented. On the other hand, attempting to keep people at home with carers beyond the time that it is bearable or safe is unethical and can be oppressive to women carers. An effective dementia care team works with users and carers and helps them decide the best time for residential or nursing home care. This process often requires a great deal of skill as the family and the person with dementia may not agree or have had a poor relationship in the past (Twigg, 1992). If the decision for institutionalisation is sooner than managers think it should be, so be it. The numbers of clients who are eventually institutionalised does not mean that a team has failed.

Conclusion

Britain needs to heal the lack of coordination between services, stop splitting off functions, and start targeting. Dementia care management doesn't need assessors, care managers, counsellors, reviewers and outside advocates. These roles can be successfully combined in the same care management team if members are skilled and specialised. There needs to be a consolidated approach to dementia care which brings together social services and health, and purchasing and providing, because that is in the best interest of the client and the family. Britain could provide a wonderful model for the world. Why doesn't it go ahead and do it?

References

Bland R (1996) On the margins: care management and dementia. In Phillips J and Penhale B (eds) *Reviewing Care Management for Older People*. London: Jessica Kingsley.

Bass D, Noelker LS and Rechlin LR (1996) The moderating influence of service use on negative caregiving consequences. *Journal of Gerontology* Social Sciences 51B(3) S121-126.

Challis D and Davies B (1986) *Case Management in Community Care*. Aldershot: Gower.

Challis D et al (1990) *Care Management in Social and Health Care*. Canterbury: PSSRU/University of Kent.

Challis D and Abendorff R (1992) *Lewisham Case Management Scheme Report to Management Group*. Discussion paper 825 PSSRU Canterbury.

Grampian Social Work Dept (1995) *Gordon Community Dementia Teams: The Health Service Component*.

Gilhooly MLM (1989) *Do services delay or prevent institutionalization of people with dementia?* Research Report 4. Stirling: Dementia Services Development Centre.

Levin E, Sinclair I and Gorbach P (1989) *Families, Services and Confusion in Old Age*. Aldershot: Gower.

Rees P and Sennett J (1992) *Social Care Worker Scheme for Elderly Mentally Infirm People and Their Carers*. Mid Glamorgan Social Services Dept.

Sturges PJ (1986) *The Interdisciplinary Outreach Team: A New Service for the Community Hospital*. Monograph, Washington DC Gerontological Society of America.

Sturges PJ (1994) Dementia care management teams in the UK. Paper presented at the second International Case Management Conference, Toronto, Canada.

Sturges PJ (1995) The Local Community as a Supportive Environment for the Frail Elderly. Unpublished doctoral dissertation, Seattle, University of Washington.

Sturges PJ (1996) Care management practice: lesson from the USA. In Clark and Lapsley (eds) *Planning and Costing Community Care*. London: Jessica Kingsley.

Sturges PJ (forthcoming, 1997) *Care Management Practice in Scotland*.

Twigg J (1992) *Carers: Research and Practice*. London: HMSO.

US Congress, Office of Technology Assessment (1987) *Loosing a Million Minds. Confronting the tragedy of Alzheimer's Disease and other Dementias (OTA-BA-323)* Washington DC Government Printing Office.

Winner M (1996) User choice, care management and people with dementia. In Phillips J and Penhale B (eds) *Reviewing Care Management for Older People.* London: Jessica Kingsley.

Weissert WG (1985) Seven reasons why it is so difficult to make community based long term care cost effective. *Health Services Research* 20 (4), 424-433.

Wistow G (1995) Aspirations and realities: community care at the crossroads. *Health and Social Care in the Community* 3(4), 227-240.

Zimmer JG, Eggert GM and Chiverton P (1990) Individual versus team case management in optimizing community care for chronically ill patients with dementia. *Journal of Ageing and Health* 2(3), 357-372.

Interventions

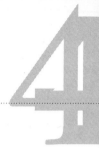

28 Therapies in old age psychiatry: reflections on recent changes

Susan M Benbow

Old age psychiatry has evolved rapidly over the past ten years and was recognised by the Department of Health as a specialty in 1989. Old age psychiatrists are now working in most districts of the United Kingdom (Benbow and Jolley, 1996), making psychiatric treatments more accessible to older people across the country. This is an idiosyncratic personal reflection on changes in psychiatric treatment and their effects on the care of older people with dementia. I make no attempt to be comprehensive, but select areas which I believe to be important, and the length of my reflections on a therapy does not necessarily correlate with its overall importance.

Drug treatments

Today clinicians have to choose between various antidepressive and antipsychotic drugs, some of which have not been available long, and experience in treating older adults with them is limited. Older adults with whom the drugs have been tried have often been highly selected, excluding the very people who are treated daily in old age psychiatry practice.

Older adults are at risk of adverse drug interactions and reactions. Physiological changes associated with ageing processes may alter pharmaco-kinetics (Leonard, 1994) and some common side-effects of psychotropic drugs are ones to which older adults are more sensitive. I remember one woman with arthritis who proudly showed me how she opened child-resistant containers with a tin-opener – not everyone has so much initiative!

Prescribing powerful drugs to older people, particularly those with cognitive impairment, is therefore a serious matter. Not prescribing them can also be serious, depriving people of treatments from which they might benefit.

Antidepressive drugs

Where dementia and depressive illness occur together, the depressive illness is likely to further impair the dementia sufferer's cognitive function and performance. The outcome of treatment for depressive illness may, however, be no worse in those with dementia than those without (Baldwin et al, 1993). People with a dementia are more likely to suffer from acute confusional states and other anti-cholinergic effects when treated with tricyclic antidepressant drugs. Newer alternatives can be considered, particularly the selective serotonin reuptake inhibitors. If people with depressive illnesses plus a dementia fail to respond to the newer drugs I believe that they should be given the chance of a more traditional treatment, ie a tricyclic antidepressant, since otherwise they may deteriorate more rapidly or move into care sooner than if their dementing illness were uncomplicated. One would treat them cautiously, starting at a low dose of a tricyclic and building up the dose gradually under close supervision, but it is no less important to treat a depressive illness in someone with a dementia than in someone with an uncomplicated depressive illness.

Mood stabilising drugs

Lithium use, its side-effects and toxicity are well established. Confusional states in association with lithium are perhaps more frequent in older adults and people with dementia may be more susceptible to them. This is not an argument for failing to treat cognitively impaired older people with lithium, but instead argues for closer supervision and monitoring. Because of the deterioration in cognitive function which a person with dementia is likely to show when they have a concurrent affective illness, avoiding further episodes may be more important than in someone without dementia. Thus a mood-stabilising drug may be considered. The OADIG (1993) study demonstrated how a tricyclic may be continued as prophyllaxis against further episodes of depressive illness: over two years dothiepin cut the relapse rate by two and a half times compared with controls.

Antipsychotic drugs

Neuroleptics control classical schizophrenic symptoms in older adults effectively, but older people may be more at risk of developing side-effects. The use of neuroleptics is less controversial when someone has delusions and hallucinations (provided these are not part of a drug-induced delirium!). More controversial is their use for various 'difficult' behaviours in association with dementias, eg agitation, restlessness, 'wandering', sexual disinhibition, hostility or aggression. McGrath and Jackson (1996) found that 24 per cent of residents in twenty-eight Glasgow nursing homes were receiving antipsychotic drugs. American guidelines recognise antipsychotics as appropriate only for psychotic disorders and organic mental syndromes associated with psychotic and non-psychotic behaviours which present a danger to the resident or others, or which interfere with providing care for the resident. According to these guidelines 88 per cent of Glasgow residents on antipsychotics were receiving the drugs inappropriately.

Electroconvulsive Therapy (ECT)

In a UK survey of old age psychiatrists 61.4 per cent regarded ECT as appropriate often or sometimes for older people with concurrent depressive illness and dementia (Benbow, 1991). Cognitive function after treatment may be better than before despite the ongoing dementing illness, because the depressive illness contributes a cognitive deficit in addition to the deficit related to the dementing illness. Successful treatment of the depressive illness can lead to improved cognitive function.

One concern about using ECT for people with a dementia is the possibility of ECT-related confusional states. These are probably more common in people with diffuse or multi-focal brain disease, and sometimes the acute confusional state can be prolonged, although its course is one of gradual improvement and recovery. Attention to technical aspects of ECT may minimise superadded confusion (Freeman, 1995). If a person fails to respond to unilateral ECT, bilateral treatment should be considered.

I have seen people with established dementias whose psychiatrists are reluctant to consider ECT as a treatment for their depressive illnesses but who have failed to respond to drug treatments. My experience is that such people can be successfully treated with ECT and my belief is that not to make the treatment available to them when indicated on clinical grounds is a form of age-related discrimination.

Psychological therapies

The myth persists that older people are not 'psychologically minded' and that they cannot change. Psychotherapies have been offered to older adults less often than to younger people. This may be related to ageist attitudes towards older people perpetuating negative stereotypes about later life and predicting inevitable decline and the impossibility of change (Itzin, 1986). Negative attitudes towards older people remain widespread in the UK, but older people are emerging as a political and economic force. The psychotherapies too have undergone remarkable changes. An important developing area is work with older adults, and field-workers believe that psychotherapy with older people can be rewarding for client and therapist. Research has been sadly lacking. Psychotherapeutic interventions do not attract the 'big money' of drug-based research. They have much to offer in terms of quality care, but are not regarded as big business, handicapping their development in relation to physical treatments.

Family therapy

Previously age has been found to be negatively correlated with the likelihood of taking part in family therapy, but this may be changing. I work with a family therapy team specialising in later life and we know of a growing literature and centres throughout the country who are developing similar work. Family work with people suffering from chronic (physical) illnesses is also pertinent to this population (particularly to dementia sufferers). Our experience has been that families coping with dementia can be helped by formal family therapy. Therapy may be an adjunct to other treatments and continue intermittently over several years, often at times of crisis, as family members cope with and adjust to their relative's progressing dementia (Benbow et al, 1993).

We work systemically in our clinic and believe this alters the relationship between family and professionals. Hoffman (1993) describes systemic therapy as moving from a hierarchical towards a collaborative relationship, setting a context for change rather than specifying particular changes. I believe we can take these ideas into old age psychiatry, fundamentally altering how we work with families, moving towards a collaborative partnership.

Other models of family therapy are also used. Research continues into the use of psychoeducational work with families of dementia sufferers, along the lines of work with the families of people with schizophrenia (Barowclough and Tarrier, 1992). Our knowledge of what these interventions can offer to dementia sufferers' families is likely to expand and, I believe, will improve the quality of care for people with dementia and their families, whether specific drug treatments for dementing illnesses are introduced or not.

Other psychotherapies

There are numerous other psychotherapies. Myers (1991) overviews the variety available in the US. Reality orientation groups are not uncommon in old age psychiatry services in the UK, nor are carer support groups, bereavement support groups and reminiscence groups. Insight orientated group psychotherapy has not been commonly used for people with a dementia, probably because such people may have difficulty in verbalising and reflecting.

Creative therapies may be particularly useful as they are not wedded to verbal skills, for example music therapy uses music to work towards therapeutic goals. Drama therapy, movement and dance are also used.

Interest in making these treatments available to older adults, including those with cognitive impairment, is increasing, particularly in the US, and this area will develop in future. Increased interest in older adults may in part relate to the expansion of the older population and increasing expectations of therapists. With the rise in 'grey power', expansion of the older population and the shift to regarding 'patients' as 'consumers' there is likely to be increasing demand for psychotherapeutic treatments.

Social treatments

As a trainee I was taught to consider treatment under three headings: physical, psychological and social. Social treatment remains an undervalued, underrecognised area. What might help a carer cope with a relative disabled by a dementia such as respite care, sitting services, home care, day care services or other interventions are regarded as social rather than medical or psychiatric. These sorts of services can minimise or avoid the use of drug treatments for challenging behaviours in individual cases. Yet there is an artificial divide between 'health' and 'social' care. I can prescribe a drug, but I can't prescribe a two-week respite break for the hard-pressed relative who might gain more from the latter. And if the relative has no break and reaches the limit of their coping ability, what has society gained but another bill for longstay care?

Old age psychiatry and dementia

Jolley (1997) writes of old age psychiatry and dementia that 'somebody cares'. I too believe that old age psychiatry is about caring, and involves making treatments available wherever possible, while supporting sufferers and their families whatever the outcome.

References

Baldwin RC, Benbow SM, Marriott A and Tomenson B (1993) Depression in old age: a reconsideration of cerebral disease in relation to outcome. *British Journal of Psychiatry* 163, 82-90.

Barrowclough C and Tarrier N (1992) *Families of Schizophrenic Patients: Cognitive Behavioural Intervention*. London: Chapman and Hall.

Benbow SM (1991) Old Age Psychiatrists' views on the use of ECT. *International Journal of Geriatric Psychiatry* 6, 317-322.

Benbow SM and Jolley DJ (1996) A specialty register: uses and limitations. *Psychiatric Bulletin* 20, 459-460.

Benbow SM, Marriott A, Morley M and Walsh S (1993) Family therapy and dementia: review and clinical experience. *International Journal of Geriatric Psychiatry* 8, 717-725.

Freeman CP (1995) *The ECT Handbook*. The Second Report of the Royal College of Psychiatrists Special Committee on ECT, Royal College of Psychiatrists, London.

Hoffman L (1993) Beyond power and control: towards a second-order family systems therapy. Chapter 1 in *Exchanging Voices a Collaborative Approach to Family Therapy*. London: Karnac Books, 10-32.

Itzin C (1986) Media images of women: the social construction of ageism and sexism. Chapter 7 in Wilkinson S (ed) *Feminist Social Psychology: Developing Theory and Practice 1. Social Psychology*. Buckingham: Open University Press, 119-134.

Jolley D (1997) Old age psychiatry and dementia: somebody cares. In Marshall M (ed) *The State of the Art in Dementia Care*. London: CPA.

Leonard B (1994) Geriatric psychopharmacology. Chapter 25 in Chiu E and Ames D (eds) *Functional Psychiatric Disorders of the Elderly*. Cambridge University Press, 427- 439.

McGrath AM and Jackson GA (1996) Survey of neuroleptic prescribing in residents of nursing homes in Glasgow. *British Medical Journal* 312, 611-612.

Myers WA (ed) (1991) *New Techniques in the Psychotherapy of Older Patients*. London: American Psychiatric Press.

Old Age Depression Interest Group (OADIG) (1993) How long should the elderly take antidepressants? A double-blind placebo-controlled study of continuation/ prophyllaxis therapy with dothiepin. *British Journal of Psychiatry* 162, 175-182.

29 Owning the past in dementia care: Creative engagement with others in the present

Faith Gibson

We talked together about our past lives – the everyday things we all remembered. We shared our feelings and our experiences and felt the better for it.
Residential worker

Within the limits of our present understanding, it is reasonable to suggest that a person with dementia finds it progressively difficult to engage confidently with others, retain a clear sense of personal identity and prevent themselves from retreating into social isolation. Both the quantity and the quality of communication between the person with dementia and others around them diminish with encroaching dementia. A failure to communicate coherently is an enormous threat to the maintenance of interpersonal relationships. It is generally accepted that dementia, of whatever kind, will sooner or later lead to language disturbance, less satisfying relationships and increasing isolation. Anything which ameliorates, retards or prevents such fundamental threats to personhood must command our attention.

Using knowledge of a person's past to hold them in present relationships is one of several creative means which can be used to maintain warm caring mutual relationships and stave off encroaching frightening retreat into isolation. Communication is a two way process, with give and take, listening, initiating talk, decoding, responding and appreciating the emotional as well as the cognitive content of words and non-verbal cues which link us with each other. Reminiscence and life history work either with very small groups or individuals, providing it is undertaken sensitively and skilfully, has much to offer people of all ages who have dementia and those who work with them.

The growing international literature on reminiscence is bedevilled by problems of conceptualisation, unsupported generalisations, non-specific studies and insufficiently rigorous evaluation from either qualitative or quantitative perspectives. Even so there is enough evidence to suggest confidently that there are many aspects of reminiscence theory, practice and research relevant to both ordinary ageing and to dementia which would repay the reader's careful attention. It is not possible here to review either this literature or to rehearse the many ways in which reminiscence work may be undertaken (Bornat, 1994; Gibson, 1994; Osborn, 1993).

Here only one particular aspect best described as a creative mixture of both art and science will be explored. It concerns using reminiscence and life history as a means of promoting conversation and conveying genuine interest, and empathetic understanding through attentive listening as the means for developing and sustaining close nurturing relationships between people with dementia and family or professional carers.

We as carers need to make ourselves as available to the person with dementia as we possibly can. We need to be able to set aside our own anxieties, which dementia invariably arouses, and our dread of being overwhelmed by the seeming irrationality of the other's condition. We need to be prepared, as best we can, to share the world of the person with dementia. Engaging in mutual reminiscence is one way of sharing this world. It conveys a sense of common humanity. If we can learn to listen, really listen, to spend time with, and to experience the other person as worthy of our attention, we can catch a glimpse of how she or he used to be and how now in the present there can still be reciprocity in relationship with each other. By exploring and sharing the long and complex journeys which people with dementia have made to reach the present, we can convey our availability as reliable dependable travelling companions in whom trust may be placed when so much else around is threatening to disintegrate.

It is crucial to demonstrate respect for the person with dementia and a belief, worked out in moment by moment interactions, in their autonomy. It is therefore never acceptable for a carer to dragoon a person into reminiscence for not everyone will wish to share their past although most are pleased to do so. Reminiscence is a recalling of everyday experience, of life as it has turned out, for good or ill, its joys and pain. Reminiscence acknowledges that we are all fellow human beings whose life stories are made and remade each time they are told to an attentive listener.

In dementia the conventional rules of communication become increasingly disrupted. Content, chronological sequence, choice of words and mode of expression are all liable to be disturbed. Emotion may become displaced and the untutored listener may respond by becoming upset and keen to set the record straight. Such listeners usually try to continue the conversation according to accepted logical rules, even if these rules are no longer being used by the person with dementia. The thoughtless listener offers interpretation, says how they think it should be said, and in this rush to correct risks reinforces the other's sense of confusion, failure and inadequacy. These mindless responses by carers may actually encourage a retreat into silence, a distancing and withdrawal least inadequacies and deficiencies be further exposed. Following each such damaging encounter there is likely to be less effort made by both to initiate, engage or persevere in conversation.

How then may the carer set conversation within safe territory in order to lessen the risk of arousing feelings of inadequacy and failure? How may carers sustain mutually satisfying talk as a means of nurturing relationships? How may the vicious downward spiral of mutual social withdrawal be prevented?

Because of the nature of cognitive difficulties associated with dementia conversation about the present, the here and now is likely to be more problematic than talk about the past. Talk about the past offers the possibility of being easier, more readily accessible and easier to sustain. It promises to be a more effective vehicle for holding people in conversation. Conversation may be about the past but it is a here and now activity and hence it offers the potential for building and sustaining relationships in the present (Buchanan and Middleton, 1995).

People with dementia retain an ability to recall the distant past, often in graphic detail, far longer than they can remember and recall the recent past. It is therefore self evident that they should find it easier to respond to another's interest in their past, if sympathetically and respectfully approached (perhaps aided by the imaginative use of multisensory highly relevant triggers to stimulate recall) than to talk about the here and now. If using this approach, carers need to acquaint themselves with both general and specific knowledge to help them locate the conversation in familiar times, places and life experience. By these means the person with dementia can be gently eased into conversation with each reminiscence in turn adding to the store of topics or themes on which future conversation may be based.

Many professional carers rely exclusively on using unplanned spontaneous opportunities for reminiscing. Such opportunities may be very fruitful and their importance should not be underestimated. Nevertheless they are no substitute for carefully planned work done on either a one to one basis or in very small groups where it is clear to all concerned that time has been set aside especially to concentrate on hearing and exchanging people's rich life experience. Small groups extend the opportunity for discovering or rediscovering common ground with peers and provide all too rare opportunities for enjoyable socialising. Specifically planned work may also result in an agreement to make a tangible record of the shared reminiscences. This record may take many forms: life story books; exhibitions; drawing family trees; tape recordings; drawings, paintings, carving, pottery or sculpture; annotated photographic records; drama, music, dance; activity projects; and intergenerational presentations (Bornat, 1994). The confidence enhancing significance of the tangible 'product' arising from the reminiscence process cannot be underestimated for the people whose lives are represented.

Providing acceptable ways of agreeing consent are achieved, memories made more accessible in some of these ways can influence not only the particular carer with whom they were first shared, but other staff, residents, relatives and neighbours. Interest can be stimulated, sympathies enlarged, new ideas about activities and occupations initiated and the linkages between the care environment and its wider social context developed. The person with dementia while becoming an active participant in his or her own growth and development is also, by these means, enabled to contribute to the larger environment in which she lives.

Reminiscent behaviour is both influenced by and influences the present context of care. It provides a sense of continuity between the past and the present and may assist a person to feel more comfortable with inevitable change. In institutional settings the older person with dementia is always subordinate to staff. Reminiscence work can only ever challenge this inequality if the staff are genuinely and honestly interested in learning from the older people and are supported by managers whose philosophy, practice and resources recognise that creative, attentive listening takes time.

To be accepted and valued as a unique person is one of our most fundamental needs. Because dementia serves to rob us of our capacity to protect this need it is imperative that dementia carers become its guardians. Our past exerts a powerfully formative influence on determining our unique personhood. If someone understands that past, even in small measure, they are more likely to understand us in the present.

As well as diminishing a person's capacity to safeguard their personhood, dementia also threatens their sense of attachment and the security inherent in assured attachments. In adulthood attachment can be achieved by self-initiated or reciprocal activities but both are likely to be seriously impaired by the disease process. People with dementia will not only have difficulty in maintaining attachment behaviour but may also become distraught by reexperiencing earlier fears of abandonment. Their present perceptual confusions related to time, place and space may mean that past attachments, now lost, may intrude into the present in troubling and troublesome ways. Furthermore, diminishing capacity to initiate and sustain conversation, especially if accompanied by distressing behaviour, may result in a failure to elicit appropriate attachment responses in carers. On the other hand being involved in acceptable conversation and associated activity with calm, stable, warm carers may serve: 'To produce sufficient interaction to foster a desired level of attachment and so reduce the sense of loss of control' (Wright, 1995, p140).

Engagement in reminiscence activity is one way of facilitating such interaction resulting in present attachment which may 'hold' the person, thereby allaying their recurring anxieties and insecurities.

Reminiscence encourages the carer to communicate as with a competent adult by showing interest, respect and responsiveness. It both confirms and uses residual ability and offers interest, warmth, reassurance and friendship. It gently demands response and interaction, without infantilism, pressure or inquisition and offers instead reduction of stress, threat, anxiety and failure. What is demanded of the carer is very complex. They have to identify with the person with dementia, share their past and hold them in relationship in the present.

> *Among the therapeutic interventions at our command, possibly the simplest one of all is the ability to listen, to accept, and to understand. A seemingly modest strategy to be sure, but one that has great implications for an improved state of well-being in the face of devastating loss.*
>
> Mills and Coleman, 1994, p216

If a person with dementia finds it easier to talk about the past, then it is obviously sensible for the carer to do the same. By listening, accepting and understanding the past, the present may become less lonely, less threatening, less devastating.

References

Bornat J (ed) (1994) *Reminiscence Reviewed*. Buckingham: Open University.

Buchanan K and Middleton D (1995) Voices of experience: talk, identity and membership in reminiscence groups. *Ageing and Society* 15(4), 457-491.

Gibson F (1994) *Reminiscence and Recall*. London: Ace.

Mills M and Coleman P (1994) Nostalgic memories in dementia case study. *International Journal of Aging and Human Development* 38 (3), 203-219.

Osborn C (1993) *Reminiscence Handbook*. London: Age Exchange.

Wright L, Hickey J, Buckwalter K and Clipp E (1995) Human development in the context of aging and chronic illness: the role of attachment in Alzheimer's disease and stroke. *International Journal of Aging and Human Development* 41(2), 133-150.

30 Neuroleptic prescribing in dementia: uses, problems and ethical issues

Graham Jackson

Introduction

Neuroleptic drugs were a major advance in psychiatry as the first effective treatment of schizophrenia. The first one, chlorpromazine, was developed in the 1950s and many others have since become available. These drugs often have dramatic effects in psychotic illness, particularly schizophrenia. There is also some benefit in patients with behavioural problems and over the past few decades this use has become widespread in two main groups: in learning disability and in cognitive impairment. However many side effects of these drugs are commoner in older people, particularly those with preexisting brain damage and evidence for other than short term benefit is weak. A meta-analysis carried out in 1990 (Schneider et al) of studies looking at neuroleptic use for behavioural disturbance associated with dementia showed only 18 per cent benefit over placebo and the studies tended to be of short duration, typically six weeks, and thus did not take account of more slowly developing side effects or of continuing benefit. Following legislation restricting neuroleptic prescribing in nursing homes in the USA, there have been various discontinuation studies which have shown that patients improve rather than deteriorate on withdrawal (Thapa et al, 1994).

Challenging behaviour in dementia

The care of older people is changing from the Victorian longstay hospitals to the 'new institutions' of nursing homes. Medical care has changed from being consultant-led to primary care-led. Staff in nursing homes are less likely than psychiatric staff to look at ways of dealing with disturbance other than resorting to drug therapy (Burns and Taube, 1990). The nursing home patient has fewer medical reviews than the hospital patient and so the need for continuing medication or development of side effects is less likely to be recognised. Having inadequate psychogeriatric input may contribute to high consumption of neuroleptic drugs; and there is often a lack of awareness that these drugs may *cause* agitation and confusion.

Many aspects of challenging behaviour experienced in the cognitively impaired in a group setting are related to social difficulties which are aggravated by their disabilities. Loss of normal inhibitions, often a feature of dementia, leads to aggressive language or other behaviour at inappropriate times. Difficulties with recognition of staff and place results in distress. Admission to hospital or a home for the elderly is accompanied by many losses – of independence, of being a householder, of a family home, perhaps of a spouse, of physical wellbeing, or of cognitive abilities. It is therefore not surprising that such patients may become difficult. Medical literature focuses mainly on drug management of such issues. Alternatives such as looking at the suitability of the placement, allowing a degree of privacy or providing appropriate activities may be of greater benefit – with less side effects (Jarrett et al, 1995). Sometimes the main issue surrounding difficult behaviour is simply one of carer understanding and tolerance.

Problems with neuroleptic drugs

Neuroleptics are valuable in the management of major mental illness. Even in schizophrenia it has been shown that patients and psychiatrists have found the side effects to be about as troubling as the illness. The psychiatrists believed that the benefits of neuroleptics outweighed the adverse effects only when costs to society were taken into account.

Many side effects of these drugs are known to be commoner in older people. There are many reasons for this: drugs are metabolised more slowly, there are lower concentrations of neuroreceptor sites in the brain, there is more polypharmacy (with risks of interactions) and there is more likely to be coexisting illness.

Conventional neuroleptics act on many different neurotransmitter systems, leading to a wide range of effects. The most important effects relate to the action on dopamine transmission, but anticholinergic and anti-adrenergic effects also cause problems. Simply being on these drugs is associated with a doubled risk of sustaining a fractured neck of femur due to falling (Yip and Cumming, 1994). Anticholinergic effects (particularly marked with thioridazine and chlorpromazine) include increased cognitive impairment.

The problems with blocking dopamine reuptake can be divided into five groups:

- Neuroleptic malignant syndrome appears to be an idiosyncratic reaction. It consists of pyrexia, muscle damage, confusion and fluctuating blood pressure. Generally it affects younger age groups, but it may be missed in older patients. Though uncommon, it is important because of a high mortality rate. It occurs soon after commencement of treatment or after a dose change;
- Acute dystonias (muscle spasms) may occur after starting neuroleptics. These often appear dramatic but respond quickly to anticholinergic drugs and are short lived. They occur mainly in younger age groups;
- Parkinsonian effects are common. They have been reported to occur in as many as 50 per cent of older patients (Avorn et al, 1994). The classical triad is of tremor, bradykinesia (slowness of movement) and rigidity. The tremor is the most easily recognised part of the syndrome, but is often absent and difficulty with walking or rising from a chair may be attributed to underlying frailty rather than to drug use. Symptoms (particularly stiffness) may respond to anticholinergics but it is usually more appropriate to stop the offending drug;
- Akathisia, or motor restlessness, is another common side effect. It can be described as an inability to be still. Onset can be from a few days to several years on the drug. It may be difficult to distinguish from agitation, particularly in those with dementia. Often patients have their dose increased, or another drug added, when this develops; an increased dose initially leads to a decrease in the symptom. Akathisia may respond to various treatments, including beta-blockers, clonazepam and benzodiazepines, but these are not always successful. Akathisia does not always remit when the causal drug is withdrawn, leaving a permanent disabling side effect;
- Tardive dyskinesia affects as many as 60 per cent of elderly people taking long-term neuroleptics (Jeste et al, 1995). There are abnormal uncontrollable movements of various muscle groups, particularly of the orofacial and upper body muscles. It may take years to develop and once established is often irreversible. Stopping the drug involved may lead to temporary worsening, while increasing the dose can lead to temporary improvement. Perhaps surprisingly, the disorder usually causes little discomfort to the patient (Wojcik et al, 1980), but is distressing for others to watch.

Ethical issues

Medical intervention in any situation requires consideration of whether or not consent has been obtained. This involves many issues, both legal and ethical (not necessarily the same). In many situations consent can be implied – that is, the fact that a patient complies with a treatment in itself indicates that he or she is giving consent. However this cannot be assumed to be the case where the individual is unable to comprehend properly – for example, where there is cognitive impairment. In order to give consent a patient must be given adequate information to make a choice, it must not be given under duress, he/she must be able to understand the information given (including the risks of taking and of not taking treatment), and the patient must possess the capacity to make a choice. The Law Commission (1993) states:

> A mentally disordered person should be considered unable to take the medical treatment decision in question if he or she is unable to understand in broad terms and simple language the basic information relevant to taking it, including information about the reasonably foreseeable consequences of taking it or failing to take it, or is unable to retain the information for long enough to take an effective decision.

Giving neuroleptics for challenging behaviour in dementia adds a further dimension to the discussion regarding consent. Although such behaviour may be a cause of distress to the patient, often referral is because of the effect it is having on carers (where it may interfere with the ability to provide effective care), on other family members or on residents in a group living situation. The issues of consent are therefore different than with other medication, such as tablets for diabetes or heart failure, where there is obvious benefit to the recipient.

If we accept that medication is an appropriate way of dealing with challenging behaviour then we must look further at the issue of informed consent. Many of those with dementia have lost judgmental ability and cannot retain information long enough to understand it or to use it to come to a rational decision. By definition, therefore, they are unable to give meaningful consent. Current practice is to administer medication unless there is active refusal, but this assumes that the patient is competent. Consent should mean that the patient has the ability to make an informed choice, not only that he or she does not refuse to comply.

Dealing with this is easier in the case of psychotic illness. Here there is clear need for medication which is effective treatment. If illness affects someone's competence or there is wilful refusal, Mental Health legislation can be invoked to ensure compliance. The concept of consent however tends to be overlooked when the patient appears to be compliant. In an important court ruling in the USA it was stated that, 'when the capacity to give consent is in question, a substituted judgement by a judge should be undertaken for the incompetent patient, even if the patient accepts treatment without objection' (Rogers v Commissioner of Health, 1993). A study carried out in teaching hospitals and nursing homes in the USA in patients with dementia found virtually no evidence of consent being sought, and few patients were felt to be able to give consent (Gurian et al, 1990).

Conclusion

There is no doubt that neuroleptics have some benefit in the management of psychotic symptoms associated with dementia – that is, the coexistence of hallucinations and delusions. Even in these situations it must be kept in mind that the elderly are particularly sensitive to the extrapyramidal and other side effects of these drugs. The drawbacks might well be more disabling than any benefit that may be gained. It is important to remember that those with dementia are often unable to give informed consent. The fact that a patient with cognitive impairment takes treatment without questioning it does not give us an automatic right to administer it. There is a need for guidelines on managing these patients ethically.

References

Avorn J, Monane M, Evritt DE, Beers MH and Fields D (1994) Clinical assessment of extrapyramidal signs in nursing home patients given antipsychotic medication. *Archives of Internal Medicine* 154 (10), 1113-1117.

Burns B and Taube C (1990) Mental health services in general medical care and in nursing homes. In Fogel BS, Furino A and Gottlieb GL (eds) *Mental Health Policy for Older Americans: Protecting Minds at Risk*. Washington DC: American Psychiatric Press, 63-84.

Gurian BS, Baker EH, Jacobson S, Lagerbom B and Watts B (1990) Informed consent for neuroleptics with elderly patients in two settings. *Journal of American Geriatrics Society* 38(1), 37-44.

Jarrett PG, Rockwood K and Mallery L (1995) Behavioural problems in nursing home residents. Safe ways to manage dementia. *Postgraduate Medicine* 97(5), 195-196.

Jeste DV, Caligiuri MP, Paulsen JS, Heaton RK, Lacro JP, Harris J, Bailey A, Fell RL and McAdams LA (1995) Risk of tardive dyskinesia in older patients. *Archives of General Psychiatry* 52, 756-765.

Law Commission (1993) Mentally incapacitated adults and decision making: medical treatment and research (Consultation Paper 129). London: HMSO.

Rogers v Commissioner of Mental Health (1983) in Informed consent for neuroleptics with elderly patients in two settings. (Gurian BS, Baker EH, Jacobson S, Lagerbom B; Watts P, 1990). *Journal of American Geriatrics Society* 38(1), 37-44.

Schneider LS, Pollock VE and Lyness SA (1990) A Metaanalysis of Controlled Trials of Neuroleptic Treatment in Dementia. *Journal of American Geriatric Society* 38, 553-563.

Thapa PB, Meador KG, Gideon P, Fought RL and Ray WA (1994) Effects of antipsychotic withdrawal in elderly nursing home residents. *Journal of American Geriatrics Society* 42, 280-286.

Wojcik JD, Gelenberg AJ, LaBrie RA and Mieske M (1980) Dyskinesia in an outpatient population. *Comprehensive Psychiatry* 21(5), 370-380.

Yip YB and Cumming RG (1994) The association between medication and falls in Australian nursing home residents. *Medical Journal of Australia* 160 (1), 14-18.

31 Technology

Stephen Judd

No other topic in dementia care is likely to get such wildly conflicting reactions as 'technology'. To some technology is a saviour, the way to paradise; others are deeply suspicious of technology and scrutinise its proponents carefully for any tell-tale marks of the Beast.

Definition

But what is technology? Part of the reason that there is so much excitement surrounding the subject is that there is confusion about what technology is and what role it plays. Most of us would not think of mains power or refrigerators or telephones or calculators or fax machines or microwave ovens as technology. But how would our grandparents have regarded such devices?

One definition of technology which may move this discussion forward is that technology is 'any tool, no matter how simple, that best meets the users' objectives'. Technology must, therefore, always serve. It must not dominate. It must be as simple as the task requires, not overly complex. It must provide the service or function that the user wants, not fulfil a function which someone else wants. It must meet the users' goals, not exceed them.

Forms of technology

Three forms of technology are increasingly being deployed in dementia care:
- computing technologies;
- communications technologies; and
- environmental technologies.

Almost all these technologies are – or should be – transparently supportive of the care which is delivered to the person with dementia.

Computing technologies

There are few computing technologies which are actually designed to be used by the person with dementia. The end user of dementia-specific computing technologies are primarily carers. These technologies are designed to expedite and structure the work of the carer and it is only indirectly that they benefit the person with dementia.

These products are typically software programs which assist in areas such as the assessment and care planning of the needs of the person with dementia and their case management. One long-established example of an assessment tool is the REPDS (Revised Elderly Persons Disability Scale) which structures the carers assessment of client need into seven categories. Such assessment tools also can provide a graphical illustration of the client's needs.

A flow-on application to appropriate client assessment is structured care planning. There are now software applications which assist the professional carer to tailor care plans for the individual needs of the person with dementia. Such care planning tools enable direct care workers to leverage the professional expertise and practical experience of others in their personal design of a care plan so that problem-solving can be fast, efficient and modular.

Communications

The increasing variety of telecommunication devices within the dementia care environment can take two forms. The first type is the personalised, vibrating and messaging pager which has supplanted the more institutional, noisy and dysfunctional nurse call systems.

The other form of communication is the 'intelligent' telephone produced by manufacturers such as Tunstall and Vitalcall. This is one of the few technology forms which currently focuses more directly upon the person with dementia. Such forms of telecommunication are prosthetic, enabling some people with dementia to maintain as much independence as possible, such as remaining within the family home or other community environment of their own choosing but with the security of round-the-clock support when they need it. Such devices can fulfil a multiplicity of needs: they provide emergency support; they can provide security assurance; and they can enable support of a reminder service.

Environmental technologies
The most significant area of technological development is the environmental area. These may be devices which are used primarily for the purposes of surveillance, control and safety.

The first generation of surveillance technologies emerged in the early 1980s and were characterised by 'closed circuit' cameras and tagging devices. The video cameras enabled the carers within a residential nursing home or other facility to observe the persons with dementia: the tagging devices, worn on the wrist, on the clothing or around the neck, set off an alarm if the wearer 'wandered' through certain doorways. While both the camera and the tagging device *may* have been an improvement upon the invasiveness of Florence Nightingale doing a round of the wards, their use today is considerably diminished. Cameras and tags continue to be used today where the duty of care is the overriding organisational philosophy and dementia is regarded as a disease to be treated. This will be more prevalent in a litigious society such as the USA. Where dementia is regarded as a disability, where there is heightened regard for personhood, then the use of cameras and tags has been seen by many as an undignified and disrespectful invasion of the privacy of the individual with dementia.

The wholesale removal of cameras and tags may make their critics feel better about the protection of rights of the person with dementia. But it does nothing to remove the concerns of the harried, challenged and overworked direct care worker. A more flexible and recent innovation in this area has been the deployment of passive infra-red systems which provide 'notification by exception'. The infra-red sensors are supported by a computer system which can be tailored to the individual profiles of the residents. Typically these systems are activated only in the evening. When used during the sleeping hours in a bedroom environment these systems will only summon a carer – via a vibrating pager – when the movement sensors have identified behaviour which is not usual, such as agitated movement or staying in the en-suite bathroom for an extended period. In the first scenario the resident may be disoriented and confused; in the second they may have fallen.

There are a number of benefits to such a system. First, unlike a video camera, it enables 'notification by exception'. This facilitates efficient use of scarce staff resources. Second, it also balances the sometimes competing demands of duty of care and the privacy of the resident. Staff do not invade privacy by 'doing rounds'. But there is a third use. The system can be used for proactive case management: the carer can identify over a period of time any behavioural developments to, say, increased incontinence and develop positive interventionist strategies.

What is in the crystal ball?

The technologies which we can expect over the next five years which are applicable for dementia care reflect developments which we will see universally:

- technologies will converge;
- successful technologies will have universal appeal; and
- the person with dementia will be empowered.

A convergence of technologies

Computers used to be little more than stand alone processors. Telephone lines were used purely for telephony. Now computers, telephony, cable and video are more and more tightly coupled together: we can sit and read electronic mail from throughout the world, send and receive faxes, conduct videoconferences and have colleagues from across the world look together at the document which we are writing. Elsewhere, as we mentioned earlier, we have computers interfacing with passive movement sensors on the one hand and then sending a signal to a pager system. This form of convergence of technologies will continue. Indeed the technology will become increasingly as easy and invisible to use as mains power.

Successful technologies will have universal appeal

Manufacturers do not produce economically for niche markets. Economic and affordable products are therefore modular, have appeal to a wide market and can be customised to specific needs. For example, any software applications which we see for the dementia care market will be – and should be – built upon industry standard platforms such as Microsoft or IBM products.

The same is true for all technologies. One of the most exciting challenges is whether we can design and equip domestic housing so that people with dementia can confidently remain in their familiar environment and that their confidence is shared by their relatives and friends. In this regard, the key issues for all older people are *safety*, *security* and *comfort* in the home. But these are issues which are of interest to all people, not just people with dementia. What this means is that the products which will enable people with dementia to remain at home for as long as possible will, in the medium to longer term, be customised versions of universally available domestic technologies. Batibus Club International is a consortium of 120 European manufacturers who are looking to develop what they call a Networked Technology Environment. They are seeking to integrate various, currently separate, systems including cable technology, energy delivery, security systems, communications systems and information technology all delivered as easily as possible. Such developments will be used by people of all ages.

What we might see emerge out of this is:

- *a house which is secure.* The doors and windows will be secured when the resident has gone to sleep – or at a time predetermined by the resident – but are unlocked when the smoke sensor is activated with an automatic page for assistance;
- *a house which is safe.* The resident will be able to select various sorts of telephones, including video phones, according to their choice. These phones can be used for normal communications, to call for assistance if they want or need it, while integrated sensors will enable the house itself to page if someone is immobile on the floor. In the kitchen ovens and stoves will heat by induction preventing burns, and turn off if the saucepan is empty. Taps in sinks and baths will turn off if they are about to overflow;
- *a house which is comfortable.* The climate and light levels will be controlled at the choice of the residents, so that predetermined levels or fluctuations of temperature and light can be set to minimise discomfort. There may be reminder systems for other personal requirements.

Most of the technology described above is already available, is not complex and only awaits the convergence of technology streams to make it a reality.

Empowering the person with dementia

A secure, safe and comfortable family home is desirable to people of all ages and all dispositions, not just people with dementia. Widespread application will make it affordable. What that will mean for the person with dementia is that they will have increased choice for longer. They will have the same choices as someone without dementia: they can stay put or they can move. Does this mean that all people with dementia will be able to 'stay put'? No, but it does mean that the numbers who today leave their own homes because they – or their relatives – lose confidence in their capacity to cope with a familiar environment which is increasingly hostile will be reduced. If that can be achieved, it will mean that a familiar environment will remain a friend, not become an enemy.

Technology, ethics and philosophy

This is not a discussion on ethics. But almost every musing on technology and dementia care includes some words of warning about 'the ethical use' of technology. Why is this so? Why is the ethical spotlight on technology when other tools, treatments and approaches utilised within dementia care escape scrutiny? Is there a degree of selectivity, if not hypocrisy, here? There is less discussion within the same circles about, say, the ethics of copyright, or the implied ethical statements of our building designs or our approach to staff education. Is this selectivity because some practitioners of dementia care are either ignorant or afraid of technology? Are they more comfortable in repositioning the debate onto the more familiar ground of ethics?

I want to suggest that we are asking the wrong question if we explore the ethical use of technology in isolation. The question should be, in my view, whether our use of technology is consistent with our underlying philosophy of care. If our philosophy values the dignity and privacy of each individual, this will determine our response to the appropriateness of different surveillance technologies, such as video cameras and passive infra-red devices. If our philosophy of care upholds the independence and autonomy of the individual, this will determine our response to different security and safety devices.

By asking such questions we can discern the ethical framework of our philosophy of care. We can then proceed with greater confidence in the ethical deployment of technology. If, of course, our philosophy of care is either not articulated or is unclear, the chances that we will use technology inappropriately or inconsistently is almost assured.

32 Life story work

Charlie Murphy and Marion Moyes

In this section we describe what life story work is. In the process we hope to refer also to reasons why life story work is important and ways in which it might be started.

Mills and Chapman (1992) speak about the difficulty of seeing 'the person behind the illness' in caring for people with dementia. That challenge is the central thrust of life story work. It concerns those aspects of the person with dementia which are important in defining their individuality and personhood now. We say 'life story' as opposed to 'life history' to consciously include contemporary aspects of the life of the individual with dementia.

In many ways life story work is the 'nearly therapy' in working with people with dementia. So many people working with the individual with dementia are aware of aspects of the person's life story however small. Yet these possibly significant pieces of information remain inside someone's head; or as a footnote to an assessment form buried in a filing cabinet; or as a scribbled note on the back of an old photograph left in the nursing home by a carer, but now at the bottom of a drawer. One of these places might just offer harassed workers the reason why Martha calls out that name each evening in such distress.

We distinguish four aspects in our definition of life story work:

- *format* – the way the life story information is made concrete;
- *content* – how the life story is illustrated;
- *impetus* – where does the idea for making this life story have its genesis – the carer, the individual, the worker;
- *use* – remembering that life story work is a tool and so how it is used is important.

Format

Readers may be familiar with the idea of *life story books* (also life history books, personal story books, personal history books). These had their origins in work with children in care. However caution should be taken against seeing a life story book as being synonymous with doing life story work. It should be regarded as one possible format for life story material.

There is a day centre in an inner city area of Glasgow which has a map on the wall of the dining room. The map is of the local area, from a time before the area was redeveloped so all the old street names are there. There are eight pins on the map representing the houses and streets where the eight day centre members were born. Stretching out from each pin is a piece of string, which ends at a sheet of A4 paper, on which there is a photograph and some writing. Some of the photographs show the day centre member, perhaps during their school years, or later on at their first job. Other photographs do not include the member, but show a place or building of significance to the member's life. The text links the photograph and the member and the street on the map. This 'octopus-like' display on the wall of this dining room in a day centre in inner city Glasgow represents *life story work*. However it is not a 'book' as such.

There are dangers in seeing life story books and life story work as the same thing – the emphasis on the concept of a 'book' might get across the wrong idea.

'Book' carries with it notions of a large amount of writing, when life story work need not involve doing much writing, only sufficient to give some detail to the illustrations. The thought of a lot of writing can in fact be a deterrent to starting the life story for many people.

'Book' also makes one think of concepts like exhaustive or comprehensive. When we think of a book we tend to feel that *everything* should be in it. This is not the case with life story. Each of us will remember and emphasise different aspects of our stories. For some it may be a special friend, an enjoyable holiday, their trade or profession, their schooldays. There is no pattern that will be rigorously followed, although there may be similarities. Certainly there will always be omissions. So there should not be a compulsion to aim for a comprehensive story. Again this could be a deterrent as someone might feel I have no material from between the wars and so get disillusioned because the life story (book?) is somehow incomplete.

'Book' also implies writing something on a subject (someone). On the one hand this can create a distance between the person helping to make the life story concrete in some fashion and the individual whose life story it is. On the other hand we speak of 'working with' someone. This is a reminder that we do life story work with the individual as opposed to on them from a distance. Hence it reinforces for us whose life story it is.

Doing a 'book' can appear like a task – similar to the project for making Christmas cards at the day centre. And like other tasks it might be forgotten about once it is completed. Yet, as we have already indicated, life story work is a tool to be used. Unfortunately there exist some projects where examples of life stories are being stored in bedside cabinets in hospital wards, with staff thinking that relatives use them on their visits and with the relatives thinking that staff make use of them to get to know their relative better!

Finally doing the 'book' can be viewed as a separate activity, where work is integral. For some it might be the case – 'it's half past two, let's spend some time on the book now'. This approach would lose out on those valuable spontaneous opportunities for reminiscence and life story work that occur in all sorts of casual interactions. Seeing the 'work' as an ongoing process will keep us alert to this.

There are a number of formats in which life story work can be presented. Some life story work is stored on a single sheet of A4 paper accompanied by one photograph.

In Falkirk there is a man with dementia living at home who has his own life story tape, although it might more accurately be called his life stories tape. The tape consists of anecdotes from this persons life retold by someone he shared these experiences with. So, for example, his brother has related an amusing event from a family holiday when the two of them saw a dog falling off the pier and causing a great consternation in the process of it being rescued. The brother came up with the idea of the tape and circulated it among his brother's friends for them to record their shared story. Consequently instead of a passive, unstimulating afternoon, someone puts the tape on, the person recognises a familiar voice, then slowly recollects segments from the familiar story and joins in with it. Again an example of life story work that doesn't depend on the book format.

From the moment that we first come into contact with someone we hear things of their life story. For the person with dementia using a service it can start with the initial assessment interview. Later on a carer may bring in some photographs from a family gathering or similar event. The person themselves may reveal important parts of their story during casual chats over a cup of tea or while clearing the table. This combination of written information on the assessment form, illustrative material such as the family photographs, and the snippets of stories and memories comprise what one might call a life story image of the person with dementia. The challenge is to come up with a suitable format for these life story images

Content

Having outlined that life story work is very much concerned with the person with dementia, in what ways can aspects of the person's life be illustrated? People usually start with photographs. There are also postcards from favourite destinations; cuttings from newspapers recalling personally significant events; and various certificates (birth, marriage, school). Tactile material should not be ignored. Some projects keep a resource box (or memory box). This might contain specific prompts for the individual or a stockpile from which suitable ones might be found. For people with memory problems a multisensory approach to communication is necessary.

It is important not to feel constrained – let the imagination flow. Anything that can elaborate, illustrate or reinforce the memories for the person with dementia can be used. In the next century we might be seeing CD-ROMS and videos as the norm!

Impetus

The life story work can begin with the person with dementia themselves. They may feel that they want something to help with their memory, or may be looking to produce a record of their experiences and the things that are important to them. A carer may want to start a life story on their relative for similar reasons or as a way of feeling directly involved in the person's care as was the case for the brother in the previous example. Workers (both paid staff and volunteers) might also choose to start the life story, perhaps as a way of starting to build up a relationship with the individual. Whoever instigates the work needs to keep in mind whose story it is.

Use

Whatever format the life story work takes, whatever it includes and whoever starts it, it is important that it is seen as a living thing and not as something to be completed and then stored away.

The life story may have a part to play at important times of change in the person's life. For example a woman who has been attending respite without any recollection of previous visits and with added distress each time may be assisted if photographs reflecting enjoyable aspects of her time there are included in a life story book. Moreover if she was able to take some of her life story material with her to the respite it might enable people there to get to know her more and improve the quality of her experience.

Similarly life story material may offer solutions to some everyday problems. Sitting down with someone and recalling achievements through a life story folder of certificates and celebratory photographs, may help someone through a despondent period in the afternoon at the day centre.

At the same time life story work should not avoid difficult subject areas; it is not simply about celebrating the past. For some people recalling a painful memory may be the first occasion that someone has listened. Often that might be all we are called to do. Workers may need to be supported through this process which can sometimes move into what is called life review (Garland, 1993).

Once started in life story work it is important to adopt a 'good practice' approach. Two points that we would leave you with in relation to this are:

- *remember whose story it is* – this should dictate what is included or not. If the individual recalls only two of his seven siblings why insist on photographs of all seven when to do so would cause distress;
- *start with belief* – this means abjuring feelings of doubt about stories, or individual recollections – very often the stories are true. One reminiscence worker spoke of her experience leading a group discussing childhood entertainment such as going to the circus. A patient piped up that he had been a lion tamer in his day. The worker looked incredulous. The member then started to unbutton his shirt – more incredulity – he was revealing his scars!

References

Garland J (1993) What Splendour. It All Coheres: life review therapy with older people. In Bornat J (ed) *Reminiscence Reviewed*. Buckingham: Open University Press.

Mills M and Chapman I (1992) Understanding the Story. *Nursing the Elderly* 4(6), 27-30.

33 What Do We Mean When We Talk about Assessment?

Gregor McWalter

Assessment is widely recognised as central to the practice of health and social care in the community. It is discussed in many texts and journals, and recent writing demonstrates the range of related issues. While assessment has always been important for the proper delivery of care, the community care reforms (DoH, 1989) reemphasised its central role and explicitly distinguished assessment from care management. These are seen as joint but distinct – together forming the 'cornerstone of high quality care' (DoH, 1989 paragraph 1.11). Central to the ethos of care in the community is the notion that services should be tailored to the needs and preferences of individuals. As a consequence the assessment of need, rather than assessment for existing services, has taken on a new and central role in health and social care in the community.

There are a variety of currently recognised problems with assessment. These include the difficulties inherent in assessing people in an equal and equitable way, of recognising the requirements of carers, and balancing these with those of the 'client' (Smale et al, 1993). The assessment of need in particular is fraught with difficulties, not least because of widespread confusion over what is meant by 'need', the lack of appropriate central guidance on this (McWalter et al, 1994; Nolan and Caldock, 1995), and the (perhaps consequent) tendency of practitioners to think in terms of services rather than needs (DoH, 1993).

Some of these problems have or are receiving attention in the literature. This has been reflected in discussions of models of assessment (eg Smale et al, 1993; Nolan and Caldock, 1995). These discussions have addressed such issues as the difficulties in assessment practice, the relationship of assessment to the subsequent management of resources, the difficulties which multidisciplinary or inter-agency working raises for assessment, and the perhaps conflicting needs of service users and carers. In addition, these discussions have introduced principles of good assessment (Nolan and Caldock, 1995).

Such issues, and the approaches to resolving them, are clearly of more than topical interest, given the acknowledgement of the vital role of assessment in health and social care. Indeed, recommendations such as those synthesised from a consideration of the literature by Nolan and Caldock (1995) are central to practice, for example that 'a good assessor will: (1) empower both the user and carer...(2) involve, rather than just inform, the user and carer...be interested in the user and carer as people'. Such principles form the manner in which any of us – professional or service user – would like to be treated if we were the subject of an assessment. They are perhaps particularly important for people with dementia, where the disease may cause a wide range of difficulties in people's ability to think, to remember, to care for themselves or to behave within the bounds expected by others.

The principles of good assessment are of clear and immediate relevance for practitioners. A detailed discussion of such principles lies outside this article, but may be found in a range of source texts and in the literature. Assessment is comprised of more than skilled practice in conducting an assessment. There are aspects of the information gathered – as well as the process of gathering that information – which are important, namely the quality of the information, in particular accuracy. This is rarely explicitly discussed in the community care literature.

The accuracy of information gathered at assessment is obviously important. Assessment is not an activity which should be conducted without a clear purpose. Indeed, 'Assessment is not something that ever stands on its own and the word should always be followed with "For what?"' (Marshall, 1990 p36). Assessment may have a range of possible purposes, for example for care planning, for monitoring, or for specific investigations such as neuropsychological testing. However, at its broadest, the purpose of assessment is to inform.

The practice of health and social care requires decision making in a variety of situations. This may include making decisions on what action to take to address individual needs, ideally in conjunction with service users and carers. In such decisions, the role of accurate information is crucial in tailoring services to meet needs. In addition, the role of accurate information as evidence in dispelling the assumptions which may form part of an assessment (Smale et al, 1993; Nolan and Caldock, 1995) is potentially very powerful.

To design services to meet needs is one current challenge for health and social care in the community. Such a task has to be addressed every day at the level of service users. In addition, it requires activity at the planning level, where services are designed and tailored for populations. One source of information generally recognised as vital for planning is information aggregated from service users. The accuracy of such information will directly affect service planning.

The adequate quality of information gathered at assessment is vital for both individual care and for service planning. However, this issue is not generally explicitly addressed in the community care literature. For example, while Nolan and Caldock (1995) make some fifteen recommendations for good assessment practice, none of these explicitly address information quality. In assessing people with dementia, gathering accurate information is often very difficult due to the nature of the disease and the effect which it may have on people. In some cases, people with dementia may simply not be aware of the extent or nature of the difficulties which they face, or even the existence of such difficulties.

To ensure accuracy in gathering assessment information requires a range of strategies, some of which may be more efficient than others. For example, direct observation will tell an assessor much in terms of the abilities and needs of their client while asking a direct question may be less effective in some circumstances. It may be necessary to seek other sources of information, for example carers, other professionals or even neighbours. This may raise ethical issues, such as discussing a person with others – perhaps without their knowledge. One difficult decision which assessors may have to make concerns balancing such ethical concerns with the need for accurate information. Assessing people with dementia is often a difficult task.

What do we mean when we talk about assessment? Consideration of these issues suggests that assessment is about more than the process of conducting assessment, more than adopting appropriate principles or even models of assessment. Assessment is both a process and a task, and that task is to gather accurate information which may be used to inform decision making – primarily at the individual level of care planning but possibly also for planning if assessment information is aggregated. The process of assessment includes such issues as relationship building, ensuring a good environment, including avoiding value judgements, keeping an open mind and being interested in the service user and carer as people (Nolan and Caldock, 1995).

The distinction between task and process is not all that assessment comprises. There are other issues, for example the distinction between assessment and care planning. Assessment is logically and theoretically distinct from the activities which comprise care planning in terms of the tasks involved – either gathering information or addressing needs. However, there are aspects of the process in each which may be highly similar, or in some circumstances even identical, for example empowering the service user and carer, being interested in them as people and listening to and valuing their opinions.

Assessment is often described as a constant activity, something which health and social care professionals are continually doing in any contact with a service user and carer. It is possible to describe assessment as either formal or informal. Formal assessments are likely to be conducted at regular intervals for specific purposes, such as to inform care planning, and should be recorded. Informal assessment is more likely to be a continuous process, where information is used for review, or to supplement formal assessment and care planning activities. In both formal and informal assessment the task is identical, gathering accurate information, although the process in each may differ depending on circumstances.

One way of helping to ensure that formal assessments gather accurate information is to use an appropriate assessment tool. These are forms which are designed to gather a specific set of information, for example about needs, disability, depression or aspects of mental function. Assessment tools are not assessments in themselves. They are an aid to the task of assessment, gathering accurate information.

There are a variety of forms available, not all of which have been fully researched and evaluated. To ensure that the information gathered by a form is of good quality it is necessary for that form to be, as a minimum, both reliable and valid (eg Peck and Shapiro, 1990). Reliability refers to the consistency of the tool, for example whether different users would get the same results with the same person. Validity refers to the ability of the tool to actually assess what it says it assesses – a good example is that a needs assessment tool should assess need and not, for example, dependency or disability. To use a tool which has not been properly evaluated for reliability and validity is to gather information of an unknown, and possibly poor, quality and accuracy.

A fully evaluated assessment form will have details supplied about reliability and validity. This may exclude many of the assessment forms developed for social care assessments under the enormous pressures of time heralded by the introduction of the community care reforms (McWalter et al, 1994). The lack of proper development and evaluation in many of the assessment *pro formas* in use may be one factor in the apparent disillusionment with such forms (Middleton, 1994, and, Baldwin and Woods, 1994, both in Nolan and Caldock, 1995; and DoH, 1993), perhaps combined with the fact that these may be confused with a full assessment in themselves. However, a properly developed assessment tool, used as part of a full, holistic assessment may be helpful in assuring the quality of the information which is gathered.

These issues are particularly important in considering needs assessments, and needs assessment tools. It has been noted that current approaches to 'needs assessments' are, in fact, more accurately described as assessments of disability, dependency, cognitive impairment (McWalter et al, 1994) or suitability for existing services (DoH, 1993). The validity of needs assessment tools may only be established with reference to a definition of need, and of needs assessment. Such a definition does exist (McWalter et al, 1994) and has been used in the development and evaluation of a tool for the assessment of need in people with dementia and their carers – the Care Needs Assessment Pack for Dementia (CarenapD).

In conclusion, the practice of assessment is a process which has at its heart the task of gathering accurate information. This may be aided by the use of appropriate assessment tools but these must be both reliable and valid.

References

Department of Health (1989) *Caring for People: Community Care in the Next Decade and Beyond*. Cm 849. London: HMSO.

Department of Health (1993) Monitoring and development: assessment special study. Joint SSI/ NHSME study of assessment pointers in five local authority areas. Department of Health, London.

Nolan M and Caldock K (1995) Assessment: identifying the barriers to good practice. *Health and Social Care in the Community* 4(2), 77-85.

McWalter G, Toner H, Corser A, Eastwood J, Marshall M and Turvey T (1994) Needs and needs assessment: their components and definitions with reference to dementia. *Health and Social Care in the Community* 2(4), 213-270.

Marshall, MT (1990) *Social Work with Old People* (second edition). London: Macmillan.

Peck DF and Shapiro CM (1990) Guidelines for the construction, selection and interpretation of measurement devices. In Peck DF and Shapiro CM (eds) *Measuring Human Problems*. Chichester: Wiley.

Smale G, Tuson G, Biehal N and Marsh P (1993) *Empowerment, Assessment, Care Management and the Skilled Worker*. London: HMSO.

Acknowledgements

Alison McWalter (Clinical Psychologist, West Lothian NHS Trust) and Hugh Toner (Head of Psychology, Fife Healthcare NHS Trust) for helpful discussions.

34 Rewriting the story of dementia: a narrative approach to psychotherapy with people with dementia

Laura J Sutton and Richard Cheston

All our lives are but a story, and this is only another. Stories should be a mirror held up to life. Sometimes those mirrors are cracked or opaque. Only those who look into it can truly know; you, the reader, will decide.

Brian Keenan (1992)

Our world is full of stories. We tell stories of heroism and valour, beauty and love. We see stories on television and on film, we read them in books and we listen to them being told by those we meet, including those people we meet who have dementia. We live in a world of stories because stories and story-telling are important.

In this chapter we look at why story-telling is important. In doing this we will be telling a story of our own about those we have been told by people with dementia. It will be a very different story from the ones that psychologists, psychiatrists and others conventionally tell about dementia which are so often about the disease and not about the person living through it.

We believe that by providing opportunities for people with dementia to tell their stories and to be listened to in psychotherapy, so we are providing them with an opportunity to make sense out of the world in which they live and to grieve the losses that they have suffered. Being able to tell a story and to listen to others telling similar stories, then, is an important part of the psychotherapeutic process.

Stories about the past are also about the present

The first thing that we need to realise about story-telling is that it is something that we all do from the earliest years of our life. One reason for this is that story-telling is a way in which we try and make sense out of our world – we try and create meaning by remembering a time in our life which was similar in some way to the present time. The telling of a story about the past can create a verbal world of metaphors and analogies, a world in which we can begin to explore what is happening to us, in which present dilemmas, uncertainties and hopes can be lived through.

A person with dementia has so much to try and make sense of. Amongst these experiences may be an overwhelming sense of loss, uncertainty and threat, all of which is lived out within the context of cognitive difficulties and a changed social world. It should therefore be no surprise that within the stories that people with dementia tell about the past we can see echoes of these losses and threats. These stories can be understood as a way of exploring the present and thus making sense out of it.

We can understand a bit more about how this process works if we look at one of the stories that one us (LS) was told in a course she ran with a co-facilitator (Julia Coombes, occupational therapist), entitled 'Making the Most of your Memory'; a metaphor itself for making the most of our memories. At the beginning of the group, participants' metaphors reflected themes of uncertainty and struggle. In stories from the First World War participants' were 'in the wars again', uncertain about the 'officers' (facilitators') ability'.

As the course progressed through the twelve weekly meetings the metaphors developed, as participants began to talk of the camaraderie that they felt had seen them through such terrible times, how the officers had done more than they had thought, and they began to talk of the time they were preparing to 'go over the top'.

Participants were on the brink of being able to talk openly about their illnesses, only to find it too painful and they drew back. As facilitators, LS and JC tried to affirm their developing camaraderie, and to accept their grief, of which their denial was a normal part, yet without colluding with the silence about dementia, both in the group and society at large.

In drawing attention to these metaphors, we are also therefore engaged in rewriting or reconstructing the story of dementia. So far this story of dementia has been largely a nihilistic one, in which Kitwood (1990) first drew attention to the experience of 'unattended dementia' wherein the lived experience of the person through a progressive neurological condition, acquired late in life, is not seen or heard. As Kitwood (1988) explains, the deterioration of mind and body that we witness as a slow process in dementia is something that will happen to us all, and is therefore likely to activate our deepest forms of angst. So we find it hard to hear the voice of the person with dementia, lest it echo our own unresolved fears (Kaplan, 1990; Sinason, 1992).

Rather it is the metaphors of the more powerful that gain voice. Baddeley (1989) for instance talks of the 'clouding of consciousness' in studies of autobiographical memory and dementia. The metaphor of a 'cloud' is a biological image speaking to the biological framing of dementia that has gained exclusivity in our time, where the discourse of memory deficit (for instance in studies of autobiographical memory) makes it hard to remember that memory 'deficits' are memory losses, with powerful emotions, to be grieved. Such discourses of pathology speak to powerful world views which make us listen one way rather than another about people. The nihilistic narrative of dementia *which is so often* retold makes us listen as though there were nothing to be heard.

Stories are told to be listened to

In rewriting the story of dementia it becomes possible to listen in a different way to the stories that people with dementia tell, in body and mind. Pat is married to Alan who has Mufti-Infarct Dementia, and we have been struck by their parallel experiences which challenge the way we think about the 'living bereavement' of dementia, commonly used to convey the experience of the carer as they bear witness to the gradual and increasing loss of identity of their loved one.

Pat would talk about how so very tired she was, and Alan said he was 'whacked'. Pat was worried about the effects of the psychotropic medication that Alan was taking. Pat would talk about how Alan couldn't even find his way about the house now, as she talked of how lost she was feeling in all this now. Later still, she went on to say how there must be something wrong with Alan's tear ducts as 'tears stream down his face'; as she said this, tears were streaming down her face. 'He's becoming a stranger to me' she said, reminiscent of Forsythe's *My Husband. The Stranger* (Forsthye, 1990).

It wasn't until after that last session that the psychologist (LS) realised what Alan had said the session before. He said that he forgot his wife's name for the first time the other day; he was losing the identity of his loved one too, and we could write a story for Alan, of his experience of 'My wife. The Stranger'. Pat and Alan were in a living bereavement together, seen and heard through the dominant biological images for Alan (of medication and medical problems with his tears ducts).

When we tell a story about ourselves, we are telling people something about ourselves, about the sort of person that we can be and have been. Sometimes the stories that people with dementia tell are of occasions in the past when they had been important people, such as a teacher, a nurse and a mother. This valued 'identity' is often in sharp contrast with their current 'identity' as dependent and often devalued people. Similarly, sometimes it seems that part of the reason for telling the story is to tell the listener that there have been times in their lives when they had looked after others. It is as if they were saying that because of this part they could now be looked after themselves (Feil, 1990; Cheston, 1996; Buchanan and Middleton, 1996). The telling of stories thus allows the narrator to present him or herself in a variety of different 'identities'.

...at a time when memory is being eroded and one's sense of who and where one is falling apart (sic), narrative provides a means of bringing the fragments together and constructing an active identity for the narrator. And the very environment around oneself, by becoming the setting for these 'life' events, becomes invested with personal meanings that support that sense of identity, of belonging

Crisp, 1995 p137

Stories need to be translated and to be respected

Listening to the stories that people with dementia tell involves hearing how they are, how they have been and how they would like to be (Anderson and Goolishan, 1988). We need to allow space for them to begin to explore what it is like to be this person and how they experience their uniquely troubled world. We need to adopt a 'not knowing' approach to counselling and psychotherapy with people with dementia in which we do not pretend to know what is *wrong* or the *matter with* them (Shotter, 1990; Anderson and Goolishan, 1988).

In terms of our work with people with dementia we have tried to listen to the underlying meaning of these stories and to reflect back to the person with dementia the nature of their feelings in a form that the person can make sense of (Stokes and Goudie, 1990). By giving expression to what is being spoken, felt or shown by an individual, and in conveying this back to the individual so it may be possible to open them up to new possibilities and refresh their existing outlook. We try, then, to listen to the emotional meaning of the stories that are told, and not just to the surface content.

Conclusion

We need to listen to the poetical, to the metaphorical aspects of the stories that people with dementia tell. But this is hard. The stories that are told, the emotional pain that can be generated is immense. When we hear these stories we need to remember that it is not just the pain of the person with dementia that we are listening to, it is not just their losses that they are speaking of; these are also our own potential losses, our own future pain. We are listening to people talking about a pain that may well one day be our own or that of our husbands, wives, fathers and mothers. We cannot make this future 'better' in the sense of taking this pain away; we can only try and listen and to help the person feel that they have been heard. This is as hard to do as it is necessary.

References

Anderson H and Goolishan HA (1988) Human systems as linguistic systems: preliminary and evolving ideas about the implications for clinical theory. *Family Process* 27(4), 371-393.

Baddeley (1989) The psychology of remembering and forgetting. In Butler T (ed) *Memory, History, Culture and the Mind*. Oxford: Blackwell.

Buchanan K and Middleton D (1995) Voices of experience: talk, identity and membership in reminiscence groups. *Ageing and Society* 15(4), 457-491.

Cheston R (1996) Stories and metaphors: talking about the past in a psychotherapy group for people with dementia, *Ageing and Society* 16(5), 579-602.

Crisp J (1995) Making sense of the stories that people with Alzheimer's tell: a journey with my mother. *Nursing Inquiry* 2, 133-140.

Feil N (1990) *Validation: The Feil Method*. Cleveland: Edward Feil Productions.

Forsythe E (1990) *My husband. The stranger*. The Independent on Sunday 3-5 June.

Kaplan ES (1990) Facing the loss of what makes us uniquely human: working with dementia patients. In Genevay B and Katz R (eds) *Counter Transference and Older Adults*. California: Sage Publications.

Keenan B (1992) *An Evil Cradling*. London: Vintage.

Kitwood T (1988) The contribution of psychology to the understanding of senile dementia. In Gearing B, Johnson M and Heller T (eds) *Mental Health Problems in Old Age*. Chichester: John Wiley.

Kitwood T (1990) Psychotherapy and dementia. *British Psychotherapy Section Newsletter* 8, 40-56.

Shotter J (1990) The social construction of remembering and forgetting. In Middleton D and Edwards D (eds) *Collective Remembering*. London: Sage.

Sinason V (1992) *Mental Handicap and the Human Condition*. London: Free Association Press.

Stokes G and Goudie F (1990) Counselling confused elderly people. In Stokes G and Goudie F (eds) *Working with Dementia*. Bicester: Winslow.

Buildings, fixtures and fittings

35 Cultural issues in designing for people with dementia

Kirsty Bennett

A person's cultural background can affect their perception of an environment, their use of space, and where they feel comfortable. Culture is a part of a person's past and present, and influences their individual character. Cultural background will influence the design of many aspects of external and internal settings, and is a particularly important element when designing for people with dementia. Key concepts such as scale, a homelike environment and familiarity, which are often adopted, will all be affected by a person's cultural background.

Some groups, for example, may prefer to sit outside rather than inside, and spend time waiting outside rather than inside. It is particularly important for some people to be able to sit and watch what is going on, who is arriving, who is participating. Some people will want to have a visual link to inside but not necessarily enter the building to communicate with others.

Some people come from cultures which have strict rules governing contact between people: who a person may associate with, and which relationships are appropriate. This can mean that the people who can use a space at any time is predetermined.

Orientation and planning can be very important as some people will need to face a certain direction, move in a certain direction, or perform certain tasks. Particular spaces, such as prayer rooms, may be required to accommodate some people's needs. Some rooms, such as a toilet facility, may not be able to be placed in certain locations or adjacent to other rooms because of the nature of the room's use. Allowance may also need to be made at entries for the removal of shoes or other garments.

Homelike environment

The concept of home is often important when designing for people with dementia. The design of a homelike environment for people with dementia is particularly challenging when designing for people of different cultures.

For many people a homelike environment emphasises a feeling of warmth and security, familiarity and independence. It is usually relatively small in scale with familiar details, minimum distances and familiar relationships. It also involves decision making and choice, and control over one's own life.

A homelike environment cannot, however, be categorised or prescribed, as it is not the same for all people and is governed by a person's cultural background, their previous experiences and their expectations.

Responding to cultural diversity

There is great cultural diversity within Australia. Traditional indigenous people, urban indigenous people, long term residents and recent migrants will see and use environments in very different ways.

It can, however, be difficult to respond to these needs, as it is usually not possible to provide a building which is to be used exclusively by one cultural group. The number of people from a particular background can be small, and the financial resources are not available to design separate accommodation for every group of people. It is therefore important when designing environments to respond to a range of cultural needs.

A case study – Alice Springs, Central Australia

The design of a new hostel for Prontier Services at Old Timers' in Alice Springs, Central Australia highlights a number of the principles which are important when designing for people with dementia from different *cultures*.[1]

Old Timers' is located on the Stuart Highway, a short distance from the town centre of Alice Springs. The site is bounded by the Todd River and nestles at the foot of Mt Blatherskite.

The hostel at Old Timers' is to be suitable for people of an Aboriginal and non-Aboriginal background. All rooms are to be able to accommodate a person of either culture, although the nature of the resident group will be changing constantly. Many Aboriginal people may prefer to stay in their own community, or may only live in the hostel for a short time.

The new hostel at Old Timers' will provide a home for twenty older people who are frail, and will also provide an opportunity for ten of these residents to live in a dementia specific facility. Each group of ten has single bedrooms which open onto a sitting area, with an ensuite bathroom and kitchenette attached to each bedroom. The sitting area is connected by a short passage to the dining room and domestic kitchen. A separate formal lounge is entered from this area. With the exception of the lounge, all the rooms open directly outside.

Key principles which have been developed in response to the cultural diversity of the potential residents are:
- privacy and community living;
- internal and external environment;
- levels of involvement in a building
- ,'neighbours' rather than 'family';
- choice;
- flexibility.

These principles have been adopted in the context of a general approach to designing for people with dementia which incorporates principles such as redundant cueing, wayfinding and orientation, familiarity, scale and security.

Privacy and community living
It should be recognised that people's concepts of privacy and community can vary widely according to their cultural background. This will impact on both the provision and the arrangement of spaces.

Privacy is not such an issue for Aboriginal people out bush where everything is settled in public. This is, however, a way of life that is not common for non-Aboriginal people and can be quite stifling for them. Aboriginal people will often draw a semicircle with a fire at its centre and spaces radiating out from this to illustrate their preferred living arrangement. This allows people to sit at the fire and share in the community, and then withdraw yet still be in touch.

Public living will be important to the older Aboriginal people so that they keep in contact with each other and with what is going on. It is important for Aboriginal people to be able to see everyone else. It is likely that these residents will prefer to use the part of the building which gives the greatest view.

Aboriginal people often don't want to be by themselves. Privacy between tribes and between men and women will, however, need to be accommodated.

The hostel has been designed so that bedrooms open onto a central sitting area which opens directly to the outside. In this way, this area can be a meeting place for people and the comings and goings of residents can be seen as they move through the building. This public space will also allow people to interact with those who may choose to sit outside around the campfire.

Bedrooms have been designed to accommodate two or more people, depending on the amount of furniture which is used.

Internal and external environment
People place different emphases on the internal and external environment and may use these spaces in different ways.

An Aboriginal person, for example, may sit in the shade of the house to get out of the sun rather than going inside. The house will be seen as an object casting a shadow, rather than as an environment which can provide protection. In winter, an Aboriginal person may use the house to seek shelter from freezing breezes, sitting outside and using the house as a windbreak while they receive warmth from an open fire and from the sun. A house is often valued as a place of security and as a place where things can be left, rather than as something which is valued for its internal *features*.

The perimeter of the hostel has been designed to provide external recesses and nooks where people can sit at different times of the day. The landscape around the building has been designed to provide a number of opportunities for people to sit outside, perhaps around a campfire or under a bough shelter. A budget for landscaping has been set aside to allow mature trees to be planted, and a range of plants and trees which are suitable for bush tucker will be included.

Levels of involvement in a building
People will wish to spend different amounts of time in the hostel. It is important to remember that for some people spending time under the shade of a large tree will be a higher priority than sitting on a nicely upholstered lounge suite.

Some people may have lived on stations around Alice Springs and spent their lives working out bush, rather than in an office. These people will be used to a fairly tough life in material terms, and will value an opportunity to be outside.

It is possible to be involved in the hostel building in different ways. For those people who prefer to be outside, it is possible to leave their rooms and sit on their verandah or under the shade of a tree, or to spend time in the sitting area, which provides an indoor/outdoor area.

For those who are more comfortable in an urban setting, they are able to move through the building toward the dining room and formal lounge and become involved in a more structured environment.

'Neighbours' rather than 'family'
While residents of different backgrounds may live side by side, it may not be appropriate to ask them to be friends or share facilities. It should be recognised that residents may not have anything in common or wish to have anything to do with their neighbour.

Given the potential cultural diversity of the residents, the design model of 'family' living in a cluster or small group which is often adopted in the design of facilities for people with dementia is not appropriate. Instead a number of units have been designed. Each bedroom in the hostel contains its own ensuite bathroom and kitchenette so that residents can live independently of each other if they wish. A front door to their unit which is linked by a path to the other parts of the building also provides opportunities for varied circulation within the building, and reduces the need to cross paths with other residents.

Choice
Choice is important to allow people to live as they wish.

In the new hostel at Alice Springs, a choice of social spaces is available so that people can choose the type of place they would like to be in: heated (or cooled), furnished with sofas and coffee tables in front of an open fire and mantelpiece with knick knacks, or alternatively similar in temperature to outside, open to the breeze, looking directly out onto the banks of the Todd River.

People are also able to choose how they move from one part of the hostel to another. Alternative ways of going from one space are provided, so that people are not obliged to be with people with whom they do not feel comfortable. (Alternatives are clearly defined through the use of strong cues such as view, colour and paving.)

Flexibility
Many Aboriginal people in Central Australia have traditional lifestyles and do not identify with buildings as non-Aboriginal people do. Areas will be used quite differently and it will be important that spaces can be appropriated by the user during their stay in the hostel. A number of non-Aboriginal residents may have spent their lives travelling and moving between station properties and will come with few possessions and a love of a simple life.

Flexibility is an essential element in the design of the hostel. As residents will come from a diverse range of experiences and backgrounds, a flexible environment will be required to ensure that their various needs are met. Rooms need to be able to be altered to suit a particular person's preferences. Alternative eating arrangements will be important, and the opportunity for people to be in different parts of the hostel according to their preference will be necessary.

Summary

There are many ways to respond to a person's cultural needs, and the environment is only one of these. It is important to recognise this area when designing for people with dementia, as it will have a direct impact on other design principles such as scale, a homelike environment and familiarity. Elements such as privacy and community, internal and external environments, choice and flexibility are key elements to consider.

The new hostel at Alice Springs will give people from a range of cultural backgrounds an opportunity to feel comfortable and to be in an environment which values them and recognises their individuality, their past and their present.

36 'A journey with Alice'

Brian J Kidd

Introduction

Lewis Carroll took Alice on a visit to Wonderland where she had a conversation with the enigmatic Cheshire Cat.

> *'Cheshire puss, would you tell me, please which way I ought to walk from here?'*
> *'That depends a good deal on where you want to get to,'*
> *said the cat.*
> *'I don't much care where,' said Alice;*
> *'Then it doesn't matter which way you walk,' said the cat.*
> *'...As long as I get somewhere,' Alice added*
> *'Oh, you're sure to do that,' said the cat.*
> *'If you only walk long enough.'*
> Carroll L, 1877

Like Alice we wander through buildings and will undoubtedly end up somewhere. But where? Sometimes it is easy to find or know our way. At other times we are confused and lost, due to either the complexity or the newness of the environment.

It is always difficult to walk in another person's shoes. Designing for people with special needs is most sensitively interpreted if we can simulate the experience or condition of the client. But how do we empathise with the experience of a person with Alzheimer's disease or a related dementia? Our best chance is to observe such people as they move in and around buildings. The problem is that each person is an individual with different responses and stages of decline.

Our brain is a device that takes in information and processes it to yield further information. When we have difficulty in receiving and processing information, we have very real difficulty in relating to the real world.

People for whom the world has become strange and unfamiliar benefit from the small scale reassurance of a known environment.

Studies in environmental psychology indicate a close relationship between the physical environment and behaviour. Howell (1980a) indicated that the physical environment affects the behaviour and the psychological states of ageing people. Gerontological research has explored the physical attributes of environments relative to individual, social and psychological aspects (Lawton and Nahemov, 1973; Lawton, 1977; Howell, 1980b).

Dementia sufferers demonstrate a general slowing down of responsiveness to environmental stimulation, increasing difficulty in interpreting important information from the environment when conflicting or background stimulation is present, and a general need for differentiation between important versus inconsequential environmental information (Hiatt, 1982). The ageing individual does not lose all ability to function, but responds to stimuli differently. Indifference and withdrawal are common to many people with confusion and may be coping strategies to adapt to a complex and confusing environment (Kidd, 1991).

Home

The dictionary defines home as the place where one lives, belongs or was born. It signifies a sense of ownership or control over one's personal environment. My own mother asserted her authority with a plate on her kitchen wall:

This is my kitchen and I'll do as I damn well like.

Homeliness signifies warmth, love and contact with others on a most intimate basis. It means the exercise of choice and a reasonable control of personal preferences such as for food, clothing, decor, furnishings, entertainment, social friendships, privacy, personal space and territory.

Home signifies a sense of autonomy and control by the individual. Many older people come from a single person household, or one shared with one partner, and they are therefore accustomed to autonomy and decision making and governing their own environment. Others enter and share this environment only by invitation. Our personal territory is so well known that we can virtually walk around in the dark, feeling confident about (say) the distance from the bedroom to the bathroom or the kitchen. It is imperative to recreate this sense of confidence, familiarity and ownership in buildings for people with special needs, for whom home may have become threatening or frustrating, and daily activities insurmountably difficult, anxious and stressful.

Alice explored the delights and the necessity for each of us to have places for solitude, regeneration, privacy and retreat. We need space between ourselves and others at times, and this can be real or fantasy, shared or secret. As children we have secret places (for example cubby houses, tree houses, under blankets and tables) and these are places to hide and dream in. As adults we still need a place to feel alone, just as on other occasions we need or seek community. Special places are essential if we are to develop a sense of belonging and attachment to home.

Think of places you go now to collect yourself, to gather strength, to think, to dream. Your ideal secret place may be indoors or outdoors, open or enclosed, intimate or exposed. We have strong feelings about and in such places. At their best they make us feel good, glad to be there, relaxed, excited or warm all over. We are drawn to these places and experience them as often as we are able. Alternatively of course, other places make us feel bad, depressed, uncomfortable, unhappy, insignificant or out of place. One of the biggest problems associated with involuntary relocation is that we leave our favourite places behind, and our ability to recreate or create anew may be denied or restricted.

In their publication *Forgetting But Not Forgotten* (Elizabeth Marshall and Dorothy Eaton, 1984) pleaded the case for familiar domestic buildings and small group sizes for people with 'special needs', involving the residents in familiar settings and achievable tasks, in buildings that blended into the community.

The idea was further developed in Australia in the mid 1980s in the Adelaide Central Mission's new nursing home units at Aldersgate Village and the Aged Cottage Homes hostel at Goolwa (both in South Australia).

Alternatives

The traditional Australian house is not always the only answer for many groups or urban locations. Consider the following:

- in the future, many people in Australia will live in inner city or inner suburban apartments or units of medium or high density. Although land costs are high in such areas, people needing specialised housing also deserve the option of remaining in their familiar neighbourhood. This will in all probability be in an apartment building, or may be a portion of a complex (as with models in Scandinavia or the Netherlands);
- specific groups, such as sisters who have lived in a religious community since their teenage years, will have a unique experience of what constitutes 'homeliness'. They may be comfortable with sharing some facilities, used

to dining together and celebrating special days. Although privacy is necessary on occasions, the sense and need of community is also strong. A different architectural response will be required;

- in our multicultural society there are many background experiences of the architectural and social organisation of a house, and these will remain important in older age. In some social and religious groups the organisation of a house plan is critical. Women of an Islamic household must be protected from the view of a visitor at the front door; kitchens may need to cater for special dietary needs or observances (for example the separation of dairy and meat preparation); the ablution areas must not be located between the bedhead and Mecca; concepts of landscaping and use of external space will vary; differing patterns of food, gender relationship and social patterns will be common;
- in one of our recent projects many of the prospective residents came from a traditionally homeless background. The typical detached house was not a part of their experience. Their neighbourhood had been the city streets and alleyways, their housing had been camps, barracks, boarding houses and short-term crisis accommodation. The solution was to respect their individuality, to provide rooms more akin to cabins and connected by *streets and lanes*;
- another of our client groups is from the deaf community. In terms of language, they are as unique as any other ethnic group, and we are at a disadvantage as we don't know their language. They also have a strong sense of social and cultural group identity. Communality is strong and unique. Special consideration of lighting is necessary to enhance their language, and visual cues substitute for aural and auditory cues. As perhaps one quarter of people in our nursing homes have profound hearing loss, we could well learn lessons from this group, and develop buildings, staffing attitudes and programmes that enhance communication.

Design criteria

The plans should respond to an operational programme of care which attempts to deal with the following cognitive and behavioural manifestations:
- extreme memory failure;
- inability to communicate;
- disorientation of time and place;
- functional difficulties in personal hygiene and habits;
- incontinence;
- wandering;

- emotional symptoms such as withdrawal, restlessness, violence, uncharacteristic behaviour;
- disconnection from a familiar environment and lifestyle.

In response to these programme goals, the building should incorporate the following principals:

- domestic scale;
- domestic detailing;
- small group size (8-10 preferred);
- clear uncomplicated plan (non-labyrinthine);
- clear and secure wandering paths;
- cues to assist in orientation, recognition and wayfinding;
- careful selection of non-agitative patterns, colours and textures;
- subtle observation;
- era appropriate design and furnishings;
- redundant (or multiple) sensory cueing;
- familiar residential rooms, outdoor areas and relationships;
- barrier-free design;
- security (in a subtle manner).

The two major approaches translating these principles are the introverted and the extroverted plan form. Both have their advocates.

- The introverted plan is one in which the key activities area is in the centre of the building, with no, or restricted access to the outside area. Total visual access is a key feature. The central activities core is surrounded by the bedrooms. The Weiss Institute at the Philadelphia Geriatric Centre is the epitome of this plan form. The CADE units in New South Wales are a variation.

  Variations of this form have an internal courtyard or atrium space, as in Minnimurra (Toowoomba) and Strathdon Dementia Unit (Melbourne). Other variations are illustrated in the Plan of Lefroy Hostel (Western Australia) and Overton Lodge (Victoria) which have internal courtyards surrounded by bedrooms, with activity rooms opening to an external courtyard.

- The alternative is the extroverted common house plan, complete with public front and private rear gardens, appropriately enclosed by acceptable fencing. These houses ideally blend into the surrounding residential complex. The key feature is familiarity of house patterns, with a small and non-intimidatory scale.

  The Uniting Church Lodge programme in Melbourne promoted this approach in the late 1970s with Regent Lodge in Elsternwick and Sefton Lodge in Hawthorn. These provided for twelve and ten residents respectively, with the kitchen as the centre piece of the plan.

In 1988 Aldersgate Village in Adelaide opened three houses, each for eight residents with dementia. This approach deliberately adopted familiar domestic forms and details, even using hedges as front fencing. The kitchen is located so as to supervise internal activities and the rear garden, and also subtly overseeing the front door. Residents can safely wander throughout the buildings and into the secure rear gardens.

Conclusion

There is no one correct solution. The success of one or another relies entirely on the commitment to and quality of the programme, and the ability of the built design to assist in this operation. What is needed is a detailed user-occupancy evaluation of each building to determine the factors necessary for guidelines for new projects, and an empathetic designer who understands the functional needs and the spiritual dimensions. The ultimate measure of success is to consider, 'If it were necessary, would I like my mother to live here?'.

In the final analysis, the building must fulfil two major roles. The first is to provide efficient functioning and the second is to appeal to sensory delights, which may in fact be the only remaining pleasure for many people. It is essential to nourish and elevate the spirit of the people who identify with the building, be they residents, staff or relatives and friends.

In our modern preoccupation with pure functionalism and rock-bottom economics we too often forget to nurture the spirit and yet this is an especially important element in frail old age, or in supported living environments.

Whatever the architectural solution, the primary criterion appears to be to present the individual with a choice, both in type and location of accommodation. One of the great tragedies of our age is that an elderly person who has led a productive and dignified life is so often forced to face the last decade or so of existence in a physical environment that contributes nothing positive to the richness of the experience of living.

References

Carroll L (1877) *Alice in Wonderland.*

Hiatt LG (1982) The physical environment and the aged. Paper delivered to Second National Conference on Long-Term Care Issues, Environmental Options for the Aged. Hillhaven Foundation and the Beverley Foundation, 1980, Washington, DC.

Howell SC (1980a) Environment and ageing. In Eisdofer C (ed) *Annual Review of Gerontology and Geriatrics.* New York: Springer.

Howell SC (1980b) Environments as hypotheses in human ageing research. In Poon LW (ed) *Aging in the 1980s.* Washington DC: American Psychological Association.

Kidd BJ (1991) Is There a Place for Confusion? In Davis C (ed) proceedings of conference Planning and Design for the Confused Elderly, Sydney, April 1991.

Lawton M (1977) The impact of the environment on ageing and behaviour. In Birren JE and Schaie KW (eds) *Handbook of the Psychology of Ageing*. New York: Van Nostrand Reinhold.

Lawton M, Powell and Nahemov L (1973) Ecology and the ageing process. In Eisdorfer and Lawton (eds) *The Psychology of Adult Development and Ageing*. Washington DC: American Psychological Association.

Marshall L and Eaton D (1984) *Forgetting but not Forgotten*. Victoria, Australia: Division of Community Services of the Uniting Church in Australia (Vic).

37 Mealtime experiences

Lesley Malone

People with dementia often lose weight and are at risk of malnourishment. A likely explanation for the weight loss is that it is due to decreased food intake resulting from a reduced ability to carry out the processes involved in eating, that is loss of the necessary motor, planning and coordination skills. When people with dementia are unable to do things they were previously capable of it is usually attributed to the progression of the disease. However, it is generally accepted that environmental factors are important and that some environments will stimulate certain behaviours, while others make behaviours harder to carry out and therefore less likely. As their dementia progresses people become increasingly reliant on their environment for cues to stimulate appetite and appropriate eating behaviour. Therefore, as many meaningful cues as possible should be used to encourage independent eating.

If we go into a restaurant we are more likely to want to eat if there are pleasant food smells than if the most pervasive smell is that of disinfectant. Supermarkets use the smell of baking bread or roasting chickens to stimulate appetite, and hence sales, and food advertising works by stimulating our senses to encourage us to want an item. Estate agents recommend brewing fresh coffee to attract potential buyers. When these notions are applied to people with dementia it is reasonable to assume that their appetite is more likely to be stimulated if there are smells of cooking prior to, and during, the mealtime. Food trolleys which arrive on a hospital ward immediately before meals are served are unlikely to provide any sensory stimulation of this type.

The food itself is very important although the types of food considered appropriate for elderly people often vary. Some hospital staff hold the view that spicy food will be unfamiliar and therefore unlikely to be eaten. Conversely, bland foods are unlikely to stimulate taste buds which have reduced sensory capacity. Individual preferences must be taken into account and are likely to be more useful than assumptions about what 'older people' will or will not like. Views also differ as to what constitutes 'finger food', but anything a person can eat with their fingers will prevent the need to be fed.

To further encourage eating the dining room should look like a place where eating is expected. Behaviour management approaches used in the treatment of eating difficulties suggest that eating should always take place in the same environment so that the cues associated with eating are strengthened for that situation, and weakened for others. Hospitals frequently do not have dining rooms which are used only for eating and rooms are often shared with other wards resulting in a rush to get the meal over as quickly as possible. Those with distinct dining rooms often have little to suggest that they are for the purpose of eating. If we were to go into a restaurant with no tables set, no menus and no smells of cooking, we would be likely to wonder if we were in the right place, yet this is what regularly faces people who are already confused. If tables could be set with table cloths, glasses, and salt and pepper, this would be more likely to trigger memories of eating. Anecdotally, people have been found to eat much better when in restaurants than when in a hospital ward, suggesting that the cues in a restaurant stimulate appropriate behaviour. Similarly, studies have demonstrated that people in hospital, apparently unable to 'entertain', have been able to provide tea and cakes when in their own home.

In general, hospitals and residential care establishments tend to be de-skilling environments where things are done for people. Safety is often cited as the reason for this, but it is also much quicker to do something for someone than to support them while they do it for themselves, even though skills are more likely to be maintained in this way. It seems that when children are learning how to do things, including eating, it often results in a mess being made but this is tolerated as a necessary part of the child's learning process. For elderly people, however, particularly those with dementia, it seems that mess is less likely to be tolerated. It is considered better for a person to wear a plastic apron than to need their clothes washed, it is better for them to be fed their meal than to spill half of it getting it to their mouths, and it is better to have no table cloths than to have to wash them after each meal. The reasons for this are clearly practical but it might be useful to consider which is more important, convenience or promoting independence. Promoting independence is often cited as an aim of care provision yet the physical environment and ward regimes in which people are operating often result in dependence and the premature loss of skills. Staffing levels are likely to be major determinants of how mealtimes are viewed and it has been suggested that while some areas of patient care have become more flexible, mealtimes still follow very rigid routines, for example food trolleys being delivered and collected at certain times.

When 'skills training' has been used with people who have eating difficulties, the use of prompts and positive reinforcement (for example praise and attention) for eating and using cutlery, has resulted in weight gain and improved eating ability. Nursing staff have also found that the use of eating aids, such as plates with dividers, plate grips, and cutlery with enlarged handles, have helped people maintain self-feeding. In one hospital ward a lady with eyesight problems was found, by chance, to eat more when her food was in a red bowl which she could see. However, many examples exist of practices which are unlikely to promote good eating behaviour or socialisation. Often support from care staff is suboptimal, for example not telling patients what it is that they are eating, infrequent communication between staff and patients, staff talking amongst themselves, standing whilst feeding people, feeding a number of people at one time and blowing on food to cool it down. Other poor practices include part-time dining rooms with patients having to be out by a certain time, narrow entrances to dining rooms, dirty tables, people eating from trays, sitting in bean bags while trying to eat, TV's blaring and missing false teeth and spectacles.

The CADE units of New South Wales are frequently cited as examples of good environmental design and practice. Mealtimes are viewed as opportunities for residents to participate in food purchase and preparation, and to promote the maintenance of related skills. All food is prepared in the unit thus there are natural smells to act as appetite stimulants. A small kitchen which may be used to make tea or coffee for visitors is available, again promoting independence and skill maintenance. Mealtimes can be varied to suit individuals and meals can be shared with relatives.

Mealtimes are obviously an important part of most people's day and apart from providing us with nourishment they tend to provide a structure around which our day is based, and an opportunity for social contact. Many studies have demonstrated increased socialisation and eating when environmental changes are made and it is hardly surprising that seating people around small tables compares favourably with sitting in rows in corridors. People with dementia have relatively few opportunities for social interaction and caregivers often have difficulty finding appropriate activities which the person can participate in. Mealtimes offer an ideal opportunity for activity and participation but one which is often neglected despite evidence that 'well-learned' activities are those most likely to be participated in. Involving the person in the meal process should be viewed as important as any of the other structured 'activities' available.

While available evidence appears to support many of the preceding arguments for what would constitute good practice, a lack of controlled research studies means that many of the suggestions for improving mealtime experiences are intuition based rather than evidence based. It would be fascinating to observe people identified as having eating difficulties, if they were to have fish and chips straight from the 'chippie', using their hands and eating out of the paper, with all the associated smells and memories likely to be evoked.

38 'You're sitting in my chair': an enquiry into the role and function of appropriate seating for the active person with dementia

Gretta Peachment

'You're sitting in my chair', he said and looked steadfastly at the offending lady. This was the first full sentence that this gentleman with dementia had said for some time. Staff were obviously surprised. Observers charting behaviour in a dementia specific nursing home were noting the behavioural variations. One lady was chair hopping. Each time there was a vacancy she took advantage of this to move one step closer to the prize, the temporary ownership of one of the new armchairs. Another variation was the gentleman who paced the corridor and stopped at the lounge entrance obviously searching for something. On seeing a chair vacant he moved in, but as he slowly lowered himself into the chair, a more ably equipped lady darted in and took the seat right from under him. He apologised and returned to the corridor to resume pacing.

These three observations occurred during the trailing of a new type of seating that was being introduced to the unit. These residents had lived in an institutional setting for varying amounts of time. All had been diagnosed with dementia, were 'at risk' active wanderers and many had behavioural problems. Their lounge room was neither particularly comfy nor cozy, and certainly the seating contributed little to the overall effect. There was the usual motley collection of chairs including low saggy ones and those old faithfuls, the high-backed, vinyl covered, height adjustable (rusted into position and not necessarily straight) models. As these people were to be transferred to a new facility designed on the lines of a cluster of domestic style houses, the opportunity arose to review the seating needs of people with dementia.

Much work had been done to gain a profile of the client base, all residents had been measured. We knew the dimensions of an average 85 year old. Foam density and the compression factors of cushions, chair stability and maneuverability, style and fabrics, ease of getting in and out of a chair, overall comfort, these had all been investigated. Confident that we had the dimensions and structural components right, we were unsure if our residents would notice the chairs and most importantly, sit longer and show less agitation. The results of the trial surprised us all.

Why were we so surprised? Two years further on, the answers now seem self-evident. Eighty-five year olds with or without dementia like to be as comfortable as the rest of us. Indeed, if you are going to spend a number of hours a day in a chair, comfort is a necessity. This is particularly the case if you are thin, bony and have a tendency to kyphosis. Alternatively, if you have the type of dementia that makes one restless, agitated and irritable, uncomfortable seating is going to increase these symptoms. Some people fit both these categories. Small wonder then that disturbances occur, that they become a nuisance to themselves, to others and to the staff when we expect them to sit in such unforgiving circumstances for any length of time.

The three examples cited above demonstrate some of the benefits of appropriate seating. First, residents who had seemed indifferent to their surroundings became selective. Teasing out what this entails highlights its significance. In terms of their dementia, there were several processes these residents went through to achieve their goals:

- a comprehension that not only was something different in their environment but that it was desirable;
- a decision made to occupy a chair. In most cases, because of the limited number of chairs available, this required a sub-plot to be planned;
- actions were initiated and followed through;
- remembrance of the chairs was retained as some came back repeatedly seeking occupancy.

Indeed the latter was borne out when the chairs were removed and transferred to the new site ahead of the residents. Restlessness and agitation were very obvious amongst those who had particularly sought out the new chairs and there was a return to a 'waiting room' type of behaviour. Second, some had articulated their requirements. This is particularly so in the case of the man who was becoming non-verbal. By supplying him with something he wanted, he had spoken a complete sentence without staff prompting.

Increased socialisation was another observable outcome. The furniture trialled was a wing-backed suite of two single chairs and one two seater settee and a shell backed suite of the same setting. Some people preferred the single chairs, others the double settees. Those who shared the settees invariably chattered to each other and it was noted that an increased level of socialisation was achieved without staff having to initiate the action. The behavioural characteristics discussed above have been observed many times over in the intervening time and in the new domestic setting. Socialisation has increased for many. The residents moved the furniture to suit their own purposes. The two seater settees are often placed facing each other so that four ladies can enjoy a chat. These two seaters have another very important function. They enable a husband and wife to sit together, to share affection, to put your arm around your partner, to hold hands or to doze with your head upon a familiar and comforting shoulder.

The houses in this new model of care are for eight or ten people. In each there are five choices of seating, two differing suites in the family room, comfortable padded dining chairs and a bedroom chair. As well there are cane chairs in the Clubhouse and outdoor settings in the garden. There are now many choices to be made.

Personal selection and choice are now part of every day. This mental exercise, which no longer involves stressors as there are more than enough chairs to go round, is a healthy activity which supports and encourages basic cognitive skills, the aim of all dementia care. Choice under these conditions is therefore empowering. To assist this process further, fabrics have been chosen with several things in mind. Confronted with two differing suites, choice is made easier and preference retained if the fabrics are not only contrasting but have distinctive tactile properties. This is particularly the case if, as so often happens, dementia is accompanied by some form of vision impairment.

Seating also plays an important role in cueing people's behaviour. Appropriate furniture tells a person what the function of a room is and what their role is within that room. A lecture theatre informs people of expected behaviour just as comfortable armchairs in an appropriate setting suggest relaxation, repose, reflection. Most residents' reactions to such cueing has been to sit considerably longer and more peacefully in one chair. This aspect of cueing for appropriate behaviour has been demonstrated to us in a unique way. Parked in the garden is an engineless car. Its role was to encourage males in washing and polishing activities. The seating/behavioural outcomes which were not anticipated were that the car would have a social role. In the afternoons two men invariably sit in the front seats and two ladies in the back!

Well thought out seating can contribute to the wellbeing of people with dementia in so many ways. Conversely, if the dimensions of that seating are inappropriate the potential benefits can be largely lost. In purchasing furniture, one should be aware that 75 per cent of people can use chairs of similar dimensions. The others are at the smaller or larger end of the spectrum. The important dimensions are seat depth, seat width, seat height, back height and armrest height.

Seat depth is important. Too short and the person has knees protruding proud of the seat and the weight bearing area is too small. Too long and the person has the cushion pushing into the back of the calves. This causes them to slump down and increases postural discomfort. Seat width affects support at the sides, too wide and this is non-existent. The person then falls to one side and in a chair without wings, people are seen slumped over the armrest. Too narrow and a person is cramped and unable to relax. Seat height measured from the floor to the top of the cushion is crucial. Too high and a person cannot have their feet flat on the floor. Again sliding forward is the only answer. Too low and the knees are flexed. The weight bearing is greatly reduced but, more importantly, this effectively reduces the person's ability to remove themselves from the chair. The chair is then a restraint. The importance of back height is to offer head support. Head support comes from the neck. A seat which pushes the head forward (as is so often the case in aircraft seating) is not offering support. The roll needs to be well positioned. Some chairs offer this roll as adjustable and detachable. Unfortunately, people with confusion are attracted to such detachability. Back height is integrally linked to backrest shape. Lumbar support needs to be positioned with care. Too low and it pushes the person forward increasing the concave arch of the lower back. In the right position, the lumbar support offers good back rest which is the main thrust of all seating, that is to offer 'rest' to the skeletal frame.

Armrests similarly should be at a height where the elbows rest comfortably and the shoulders are not unnaturally raised. The front of the armrest, however, needs to be raised a little. This is to support the action of raising oneself from the chair. One needs to maximise the support of the upper limbs in positioning to the body to attain an independent, upright position.

The aim of good seating is to be enabling, inappropriate dimensions can be disabling. When the latter occurs, the resident may need unnecessary assistance to lower him/herself into a chair, or be unable to get enough leverage to rise unaided. In the latter case the chair, as mentioned above, effectively becomes a restraint. This entails all the problems associated with such restrictions, increased agitation, calling out, disorientation, a propensity to falls and increased incontinence.

Any discussion of seating for people with dementia cannot be divorced from the facilities continence programme. The use of continence diaries and the role of continence aids means that, in terms of seating, dampness, not flooding, is the issue with which one must contend. With an appropriate inner liner which restricts the absorption of moisture but still allows air to move in and out of the cushion, and clear cleaning instructions for staff, this is not a major problem. In fact, it has been observed that good seating can aid continence. When comfort is assured and staff note restlessness developing, it is a cue for them that there is a need for the person to be toiletted.

Seating is one aspect of the built environment which, if effectively managed, can contribute substantially to the person with dementia's sense of wellbeing. By promoting independence and function, by cueing for appropriate behaviour offering visual and tactile stimulation, encouraging choice in a non-stressful manner, creating opportunities for appropriate socialisation and lastly offering comfort and rest, seating is a powerful tool often overlooked but rich in potential.

Note

A fuller discussion of this topic, including measurements, is available in *Guidelines for the Purchase of Lounge, Dining and Occasional Chairs for Elderly Longterm Residents* by Janet Wagland and Gretta Peachment, published by the Dementia Services Development Centre, University of Stirling.

References

Christenson M (1990) Ageing, the designed environment (chair design and selection for older adults). *Physiotherapy and Occupational Therapy in Geriatrics* 8(3/4), 67-131.

Finlay OE, Boyles JB, Rosen C and Milling J (1983) Effects of chair design, age and cognitive status on mobility. *Age and Aging* 12, 329-335.

Training

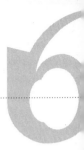

39 Is multidisciplinary training possible?

Alan Chapman

Providing effective community based health and social care within local areas for people with dementia and their families, and changing views about how services should be delivered, have led to radical and rapid changes for many professionals. Care in the community means that institutional care is seen as a less desirable option and so staff are redeployed out of hospitals or residential homes. The community nurse, the occupational therapist, the community social worker and the general practitioner are forced to work closer together as funding becomes linked to the efficient use of local resources. Consequently senior managers of health and welfare agencies have been propelled into collaborative community based dementia projects. Many of these adopt a multidisciplinary team approach to the provision of services.

Multidisciplinary teams are in vogue. Working well, such teams can constructively address conflicts and can benefit from the diversity of perceptions and the particular skills of individual team members. But what happens when the team for some reason does not work or does not achieve the outcomes set by senior mangers? How do you encourage team members to be creative and innovative when their prior experience has been to stifle their creativity? What can be done to make teams gel and benefit from the variety and richness of experience?

The answer to such questions is often a multidisciplinary training course. The identified training requirements are stated as 'the team need to understand more about the special needs of people with dementia'. Although this is an important knowledge base the training agenda for teams, as I have recently discovered, can be radically different from the manager's perception.

As a specialist trainer I am called in by managers to lead inter-agency dementia courses for groups of staff. Despite all the time spent on consultation and personal preparation I still meet participants who are angry and frustrated at being sent on training. Others express disappointment and dissatisfaction that the course did not fulfil their expectations. Such negative responses are usually offset by those who are highly motivated. The question is: 'Is multidisciplinary training possible?'

This chapter explores why multidisciplinary training is problematic and makes suggestions as to how it can be made more effective. I feel that some fundamental aspects about multidisciplinary training are being ignored by managers and that team members come with conflicting expectations.

Conflicting expectations

These differing expectations of training are influenced by the acquired baggage of skills, values, attitudes, and life experience of each team member. For those who have had a professional course of study there is an added value system associated with the role they perform. An example from a project for the training of general practitioners was that their approach to learning has been dictated by the need to identify symptoms and treatments for particular illnesses. This is not necessarily inappropriate but becomes a barrier to the use of experiential methods of learning which seeks to encourage more creative strategies. Professional training seems to have the effect of closing people off to thinking differently about shared values and approaches to situations. McMichael (1995) identified from her research how teachers and social workers had similar values and ideas about particular situations prior to starting their respective professional courses. Significantly, after qualification, they had moved further apart. Each group had adopted stereotypical attitudes towards the other and consequently were much more prepared to identify what the other professional should do.

Despite an explicit agenda about new learning, the implicit agenda is often about protection of professional status. At a recent multidisciplinary training session with a multidisciplinary team this phenomenon was evident. The occupational therapists felt their unique skills were not being fully utilised by the rest of the team. At the same time the social workers felt that their unique assessment skills were being devalued by the inclusion of the occupational therapists. A comment from the occupational therapists that the training was teaching them nothing new was a sentiment that *had* to be echoed by the social workers in the room. Significantly it was the unqualified worker in the team who was motivated and prepared to participate in thinking through the issues and reflect on actual practice.

Engaging teams in training requires an expectation that a process of learning will take place. The team that demands a lecture rather than a planned experiential workshop gives a clear message to the trainer. Flight from the crucial task of exploring whether some problems exist because of team disfunctioning, or a defensive stance because of other pressures. Learning is more than gaining knowledge. This is no substitute for the process of individual reflection on practice and applying new learning to practice situations.

If teams can have a narrow view of training then so often do managers. Training, for too long, has been regarded as an ad hoc one-off session, usually when a crisis arises or change is necessary. Participants are required to attend, made aware of the concerns of senior mangers and then expected to go out and implement the change with no further training organised. The course is used to remedy the lack of strategic planning or the feelings of chaos when too much change has occurred over a short space of time. The expectation is that the experience will remedy the ills of staff who are feeling devalued, demoralised and dispirited. In these circumstances there can be discrete organisational phenomena: the leaders and heroes, myths and legends, beliefs, values and attitudes, rites and rituals which combine to act as barriers to change and application of new learning to practice. Many teams have a sense of helplessness and training can confirm the powerful influence of the predominant culture on their practice. They sometimes subscribe to the ideas of leaders and heroes, 'Oh yes our previous Director really knew about the job...she always consulted and talked with the staff and you knew what was expected.'

If training is to be the staff dimension of service development then it has to be an ongoing integral part of any strategic thinking. More crucially an understanding of what is meant by training is required.

What is training?

A colleague training officer reflected one view of training when she told me: 'It is more efficient and time saving to tell people the answers rather than prolong things by participative discussion groups.'

This narrow mechanistic view of training has to be challenged. Participants on training bring a richness of experience and have potential for change but need to be engaged. Honey (1996) in a recent article highlights that training should be seen as a means to engage individuals in a learning process. In other words a process where people *do, review, conclude and plan*. Learning is then a continuous process grounded in the reality of experience. Consequently when we think about training for mixed groups of staff working with people with dementia and their carers, the approach has to be one which begins with what the individual brings to that situation. The training course becomes the means whereby individuals take time to reflect on their concerns, acknowledge their different value systems, discover important problems and questions and seek to develop answers.

When no explicit reference is made to this learning process it is assumed that people will learn what the manager or trainer wants them to learn. Downs

(1994) gives the warning that, 'Training does not always bring about the right type of learning and that people learn in spite of the training they receive.' Here lies the danger. Those who come on training are influenced more by the actual reality of practice rather than theoretical constructs or important facts. To use a training session only to focus on abstract concepts and principles for practice fails to address the fact that we all learn differently and the application of new learning to practice has to fit in with how each team member perceives the situation. A training course is a means to empower the individual to set the agenda and passes some control for the learning to each individual. Such a view of training seeks to work in partnership with those attending and leaves each individual with a responsibility for what they learn.

The components of effective multidisciplinary training

Engaging teams in a learning process begins with gaining a better understanding of each others' professional systems, culture, roles and responsibilities. The tribal nature of the professionals means that face to face contact is crucial. Consequently in addition to any special training event local contacts should occur, perhaps on some local area issue or a regular lunchtime meeting to discuss particular client cases. This talking about common concerns can be further facilitated by agreeing on exchange visits, for example, where the general practitioner spends a morning with the social worker and the social worker spends time at the practice; a simple suggestion but one that is rarely considered. It can apply to all the primary care team members. It certainly will involve the use of skills of negotiation and adopting a non-confrontational response.

Be clear about the shared curriculum

Dementia as an illness is a feature of the workload of many professionals. Working with people with dementia and their carers requires staff to demonstrate skills. The changing effect of the illness on the person and the anxiety and insecurities it causes requires workers to have the ability to communicate and establish relationships. They must be effective problem-solvers who can take a large amount of responsibility for people in complex circumstances. They also need to be able to deal with their own stress.

Potentially this stress tempts different professionals to come together to tackle the thorny issues of how they work together to provide effective support. When planning multidisciplinary training it is tempting to try to create the ideal cohesive team. Given the different training experiences of professional groups an alternative approach is often desirable.

A problem-solving approach is one alternative. The training agenda is set by the problems and issues that the different professionals share. For example, in the community care of people with dementia, assessment is often a major difficulty. Different professional groups want an assessment tool that can simplify their work and end the multiplicity of assessments that are done. Adopting a problem solving approach means that the explicit purpose of the training is to enable the team to find solutions. Rather than teach the trainer helps participants to use practice experiences to identify why that issue presents such a difficulty. It does not end professional rivalries but promotes the view that each professional discipline has a unique contribution to make to the team.

Create opportunities to apply learning to practice

Learning has to be supported. The learning process recognises that some change might need to take place in working practice. Both managers and teams need to create opportunities for new learning to be tried and tested.

As an example there is little point in considering a new inter-agency community based assessment format if only one professional group consider it worth following through. One method of ensuring the application would be to set up a short term (less than three months) pilot project. All staff would begin to use the new form in practice. As part of this process an external facilitator, who could be the trainer, meets with the group to review progress and identify the factors that are required to sustain it.

Conclusion

There is a role for multidisciplinary training if there is a willingness and motivation by all the professionals involved to acknowledge that there is an interdependence on each other. As the pressures grow for the effective use and sharing of resources such training sessions will become more frequent. However the key to any successful application of learning is a culture of the organisation which allows for mistakes and for individuals to learn from them. This requires an ongoing commitment by managers and teams to communicate and look at ways of introducing a training focus into supervision meetings, focused group discussions and organising inter-professional forums on dementia issues.

References

Downs S (1994) Developing learning skills in vocational learning. In Thorpe M, Edwards R and Hanson A (eds) *The Culture and Processes of Adult Learning*. London: Open University/Routledge.

Honey P (1996) What's in a name? *Training Officer Journal*, March 1996.

McMichael P (1995) Tribalism and other explanations of inter-professional conflict, paper in *Peacemaking Between the Tribes*. Stirling: Dementia Services Development Centre.

40 Sir James Mccusker Training Foundation: developing a dementia care consultancy service

Beth Douglas

The Sir James Mccusker Training Project is the dementia specific training arm of Anglican Homes in Perth, Western Australia. The project was established in 1990 through the generosity of Sir James Mccusker and his family. The training developed by the project is based on the philosophy of care practised in the dementia specific Lefroy Hostel. The founding father of this philosophy of care was Dr Richard Lefroy.

In 1994, the then Commonwealth Department of Human Services and Health in Australia provided a grant to the Sir James Mccusker Training Project (SJMTP) to facilitate an Outreach Demonstration Project (ODP). The purpose of this project was to demonstrate how the Lefroy Hostel philosophy of care could be fulfilled in other residential care settings. This was part of the five year National Action Plan for Dementia Care.

The aim of the ODP was to provide a consultancy service that would demonstrate to hostel and nursing home staff a methodical approach to problem solving issues of concern for specific residents. The consultancy service was conducted by a registered nurse and/or an occupational therapist. The major element of the consultancy was a three-hour workshop with the hostel or nursing home staff involved with the care of a specific person with dementia.

The objectives of the consultancy were to enable the staff to: effectively manage a particular situation; transfer these skills to other situations; identify their own good practice; reduce the intensity/frequency/effect of behaviours identified by the staff as difficult; and provide recommendations to the hostel or nursing home regarding management of complex situations which may be outside the scope of the facility.

The project was funded for twelve consultancies. A brochure informing nursing homes and hostels of the service was sent to over 200 facilities throughout Western Australia. Forty-six applications were received. The selection process involved distributing the allocated places between country and city locations, and between nursing homes and hostels.

The selected nursing homes and hostels were contacted by telephone to ascertain: the name of the contact person; that the identified resident had a documented diagnosis of dementia; that the family were aware of the diagnosis of dementia and that the family were in agreement with the current problem being presented to the consultancy; and that the hostel or nursing home management would encourage staff to attend the three-hour workshop.

After the telephone contact, a questionnaire was forwarded to the nursing home or hostel. The purpose of the questionnaire was to gather information on the person's past social/medical history; the current problem; current levels of functioning and recent past and current medications. The content of the three-hour workshop was based on this information.

Handout material and worksheets for the workshop were selected according to the needs of the particular person with dementia. In some instances, a video about dementia and/or the specific identified issue was sent to the nursing homes/hostel for the care team to view prior to the three-hour workshop.

A date was set for the three-hour workshop. On the day of the workshop, if appropriate, the consultant spent a half hour with the resident before meeting with the staff. The meeting with the resident was informal and friendly and enabled the consultant to see the person in their usual environment.

Two example case studies explain the discussions that took place during the workshops. A set of symbols was used that enabled staff to consider systematically the resident's needs and abilities, and what could and could not be changed.

After each workshop, at least one follow-up telephone call was made by the consultant to the nursing home or hostel to gather information about the progress for the person with dementia, the family and the staff. If required, further relevant literature and/or video tapes were sent to the nursing home/ hostel to enable staff to continue learning.

One month after the follow-up workshop, two questionnaires were sent to the service provider. The first questionnaire was filled out by the contact person; the second questionnaire was filled out individually by the staff who attended the workshop.

The final report on the ODP concluded that overall the objectives of the consultancy were met. Staff were able to problem solve for particular situations; make specific changes to care practices; identify their own good practice; and, in some situations, reduce the intensity and frequency of behaviours that were identified as difficult. This can be seen in case study 1.

For some case studies, staff stated in the follow-up questionnaire that although nothing changed for the client, the staff themselves felt differently about the client or family. This is demonstrated in case study 2.

Since the completion of the case studies, the project has continued to deliver the consultancy service to nursing homes and hostels throughout Western Australia. The result has been that, in the three-hour workshop, effective care has been planned for specific residents, and staff receive dementia care training.

Case Study 1

Background

Mr Brown, who is 82 years old, lives in a hostel. He has a diagnosis of dementia and his current problems are a high level of anxiety and reduced intake of diet and fluids. On meeting Mr Brown, he was neatly groomed, unable to sit or stand for very long and was constantly pacing. He engaged in short disjointed dialogue about the present and more detailed dialogue about the past.

Intervention

All twelve direct care staff from the hostel attended the workshop and expressed their own feelings of inadequacy in dealing with Mr Brown's anxiety.

A set of pictorial symbols was used that enabled the staff to identify that Mr Brown has physical, social, emotional, cognitive and spiritual aspects to his being. Through the symbols the staff also identified his need to feel secure, comfortable, connected to his surroundings, satisfaction and pleasure. Furthermore, discussion took place on his need to feel secure, comfortable and connected to his surroundings first, before he could experience satisfaction and pleasure.

The workshop participants used the symbols to recognise that Mr Brown had a past; was living in the present; and that his future needs required careful consideration, before planning how to provide care.

The participants also identified that Mr Brown could take information in through the senses of physical touch, sight, hearing, taste and smell. This gave the staff a sense of increased pathways to communicate with Mr Brown rather than just through using words.

Discussion took place on how Mr Brown spent his time. Staff explained how his day began. Frequently staff woke Mr Brown for breakfast at 8.00am. The facilitator asked why this was necessary. At first staff felt it was necessary to wake him for breakfast because of his low dietary and fluid intake. Participants later decided that he could be left to sleep and wake naturally, and they would monitor the outcome.

Outcome

Over the next ten days staff stopped waking the client, and Mr Brown sometimes slept until 11.00am. His anxiety level dropped significantly and staff felt more comfortable in providing care to Mr Brown.

Hostel staff were able to identify their own good practice, and with increased knowledge, they were able to change the structure of their day, in a way that met Mr Brown's needs. Two months after the workshop, Mr Brown's weight had increased. He was spending time sitting listening to music, enjoying the company of others, looking forward to his meals, as well as going for leisurely walks in the garden.

Case Study 2

Background
Mr Green is 88 years of age, lives in a hostel and has a diagnosis of dementia.

The problems presented to the ODP were aggression, and constantly asking for and looking for his family. There was considerable tension between the staff and Mr Green's son over issues such as his bringing in sweet food for his father at mealtime, and not arriving to take Mr Green on prearranged outings.

Intervention
Twelve staff members participated in the workshop. The family were invited to attend the workshop. The son who was experiencing conflict with the staff attended the workshop.

At the commencement of the workshop the staff expressed feelings of indecision and frustration in caring for Mr Green. These responses were written down, and were not revealed to the son. Throughout the workshop both the son and the staff were invited to contribute their thoughts.

A set of symbols were used as a framework for the workshop.

The areas identified for possible change were for the staff to see Mr Green in his wholeness. This was done using a symbol to demonstrate that Mr Green had physical, cognitive, social, emotional and spiritual needs. Staff also identified a greater recognition was needed of past, present and future aspects of Mr Green's life.

The need for specific communication skills was discussed. Staff recognised the need for eye contact, eye level, simple words and simple sentences.

Staff also discussed their need to recognise the impact the move into the hostel had on both Mr Green and his son. They had lived together for the past thirty years.

The son recognised the need for him not to bring cake to the hostel for his father, just before the midday meal, and the need to tell his father in advance if he could not take him on their regular Wednesday outing.

The staff also recognised that the aggression sometimes seen in Mr Green is not 'bad behaviour', but a man with dementia coping the best way he could in a world he couldn't always understand.

Outcome

At the end of the workshop staff said they had identified helpful aspects of the care they were giving Mr Green. They also said they could see both Mr Green and his son as people, rather than 'just a resident' and 'just a son'.

The son said he felt 'privileged to be part of the workshop' and that his understanding of both his father and the staff had been expanded.

When the facilitator met with a staff member several weeks after the workshop, the staff member commented 'it's amazing how the son has changed'. The facilitator believes that part of that change also occurred within the staff, but was not recognised by them. The contact person from the hostel said that something had changed because Mr Green and his son were happier, but she could not identify what had changed.

Younger people with dementia

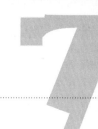

41 Younger people with dementia: challenging the system

Sylvia Cox

The way that particular diseases and disabilities are seen and interpreted by wider society is related to the way they are treated in the community and to the extent of their visibility in the media. Asked to think about their image of someone with dementia, people do not tend to think of a 45 year old man suffering from Alzheimer's with a wife and teenage children and a business to run, or a 25 year old mother with AIDS. Situations such as these often remain hidden.

Medically speaking people under 65 with dementia are referred to as cases of 'early onset' dementia. It is somewhat confusing in that 'early onset' is sometimes understood to be the early stages of dementia no matter what the age of the person, rather than dementia among younger age groups. This would not matter quite so much if everyone was responded to in an individualised way irrespective of their age. Unfortunately, however, health and social care services, funding arrangements, professional expertise, service programmes and projects have all tended to perpetuate this arbritrary division. Thus, it is suggested here, 'younger people with dementia' would be a more helpful descriptive term. However even this term includes a wider range than most people realise. Many will be aware that Alzheimer's disease can occur earlier in life, but there are numerous other dementias which exist on their own or along with other diseases. Here are some examples of the range of problems that can then arise:

- what about someone with AIDS who develops dementia? Who is the expert – the consultant in HIV or the psycho-geriatrician? Does the person with dementia stay at the day centre or hospice with other people with HIV/AIDS or is (s)he admitted to a longstay ward for older people or those with psychiatric illness?

- what about a 50 year old with Downs Syndrome living in a supported housing unit, who has now been diagnosed as having dementia? Should this person be cared for in their home, go back to live with their frail parents or be admitted to a nursing home for older people?
- who helps the family whose truanting teenage daughter has to stay at home to care for her family because her mother has Pick's Disease and her father needs to work?

When it comes to research and evaluation of developments in practice younger people with dementia have been a relatively neglected group compared with older people despite the fact that the pioneering work of Alzheimer himself was based on people in their fifties (Alzheimer, 1907). The need for research to assist multi-agency practice in this area has been highlighted (Cox and McLennan, 1994; Keady and Nolan, 1994).

A range of recent studies have highlighted some positive innovative developments but on the whole have confirmed continuing carer and user dissatisfaction with existing resources – mainly a case of too little too late (Delaney and Rosenvinge, 1995; Newens et al, 1995; Sperlinger and Furst, 1994; Quinn, 1996). Many younger people with dementia and their carers have not been prepared to utilise what they see as inappropriate day, respite and home care services. Other problems identified have included delays in being given a diagnosis, lack of advice and counselling following the diagnosis and poor community support services.

There still appears to be ambivalence, particularly on the part of policy makers, planners and practitioners in health and social care as to how to address the problem. Why is this? The range of need and relatively small numbers are obviously relevant (the Alzheimer's Disease Society have estimated that there are 636,000 people with dementia in the UK, which includes approximately 17,000 people with younger onset dementia (ADS, 1995).

Diversity and equity are difficult problems for health and social care systems to manage but perhaps there are more fundamental reasons for this neglect. Featherstone and Hepworth (1993) describe the images of ageing in our society which present fearful stereotypes of senility including the process of infantilisation described by Hockey and James (1993). When dementia appears in younger people it is as if the nightmare has become a reality: what was hoped to be postponed, if not avoided, happens at a much earlier stage than expected, shattering the life plans, hopes and expectations cruelly before time. However, many people will live for a number of years before reaching the terminal stage. The quality of their life and the wellbeing of carers and families is thus an important consideration.

Why are the needs and problems of younger people different?

The argument is not that younger people deserve better or more extensive services than older people rather that they, their partners and families have overlapping but different needs and problems to those of older people. These differences have to do with:

- life stage – past life history and current roles, responsibilities and concerns;
- lifestyle – what people see as significant and important in their lives;
- coping reactions and solutions;
- retained mobility and physical strength;
- the importance of dependant children – from babies to teenagers;
- the work role may be more significant;
- financial commitments and concerns;
- genetic issues arising from diagnosis;
- family, friends and wider society expectations about appropriate and acceptable behaviour;
- wider social contacts and networks;
- perspectives on loss, the prospect of death and on the meaning of their condition;
- expectations of ordinary everyday life – work, money, social and sexual relationships, independence and responsibility for others;
- more likely to be living in ordinary housing rather than hospital or institutional care;
- will have a different body image.

Clearly these factors are not exclusive to younger people but taken together will have a significant impact on the way that dementia is experienced by the person and their social network.

Because of the reasons summarised in the previous section many of these differences have only been partially dealt with in recent and current practice. Therefore the present state of the art leaves something to be desired.

There are some positive features in recent developments in current practice which could be built upon to develop a more coherent and positive approach to the treatment and care of younger people with dementia, their partners and families.

Person-centred approaches

Person-centred planning (O'Brien 1993) in the broadest sense is a reaction against institutionalised and service-led approaches It is also an assertion of the centrality of the needs of the person with dementia which promotes a psychosocial rather than biomedical view (Kitwood, 1993). Many of the developments for younger people in relation to lifestyle and age-appropriate day activities, clubs, use of ordinary community facilities such as swimmimg pools and gymnasiums, pubs and clubs, incorporate this approach. Attempts to provide companions for people to enable them to continue existing activities and interests both within the home and going into the community, provide more satisfactory experiences for the person and acceptable respite for the carer. Such models can respond more appropriately to language and cultural differences as experienced in black and ethnic minority communities (Ahmad, 1990). Other initiatives are transferring models of supported employment to people with dementia, offering both support in existing job locations and finding and supporting people in new jobs.

Multidisciplinary working

In many locations different staff in specialities such as psychiatry, neurology, psychology, nursing, social work, HIV, drug and alcohol dependancy, learning disability are working much more closely together. Often this has been built up through informal networks but it is sometimes facilitated by the setting up of community mental health teams which include people with dementia of all ages. This answers one of the problems of users and carers in terms of access to diagnosis and services – a 'one door' approach and clear pathways to service. Other developments have gone much further offering integrated dignostic, psychosocial and carer support and services.

There are still very many areas which are only developing very slowly. These include a much more developed and integrated approach to the needs of children and teenagers, particularly in ensuring that they are given emotional support using either individual, group or family counselling and not exploited inappropriately as carers because of inadequate community health and social services (Robertson, 1996).

Counselling and psychotherapy services similarly, although beginning to be developed, have considerable scope for expansion particularly in relation to groupwork (Yale, 1995).

The creation of positive alternatives to hospital and longstay nursing home care in the form of small-scale domestic accommodation in the community is only just developing and mainly in the field of respite care. However, housing alternatives which include partners and children are also being considered. Palliative and hospice care approaches are beginning to be developed based on experience in the cancer and HIV/AIDS fields, involving both outreach and residential care (Wilson et al, 1996).

Younger people with dementia will have different expectations and needs in relation to the design of respite and longstay facilities: they need space and facilities which promote ongoing contact and intimacy with partners and children; lifestyle expectations will affect preferences in layout, furniture and fittings, televisual and music facilities and opportunities for physical activity. Computerised systems for accessing and controlling the environment may be more familiar and achievable for younger people.

The diversity and complexity of the types of dementia which may affect younger people has led to fragmentation of services and marginalisation of needs. This should not disguise the fact that many of the problems experienced by younger people with dementia and their families, no matter the cause, may be very similar. The fields of learning disability, Alzheimer's, HIV/AIDS, brain injury and other specialties, have developed their own areas of understanding, techniques, expertise and service developments and in so doing opened up a potentially enormous range of solutions and innovations. Some of these developments have been set out and other areas identified. One of the key factors is the boundary between professional specialties, health and social care systems which must continue to become more open to exchange and collaboration. With determination, cooperation, the creative use of existing resources and some additional investment, solutions can be found.

References

Ahmad B (1990) *Black Perspectives in Social Work*. Birmingham:Venture Press for Race equality Unit/National Institute for Social Work.

Alzheimer A (1907) On a peculiar disease of the outer brain. English translation. *Psychiatry and General Medicine* 63, 146-148.

Alzheimer's Disease Society (1995) *Services for Younger People with Dementia*. London: Alzheimer's Disease Society.

Cox SM and McLennan JM (1994) *A Guide to Early Onset Dementia*. Stirling: Dementia Services Development Centre.

Delaney N aand Rosenvinge H (1995) Presenile dementia: sufferers, carers and services. *International Journal of Geriatric Psychiatry* 10, 597-601.

Featherstone M and Hepworth M (1993) Images of ageing. In Bond J, Coleman P and Peace S (eds) *Ageing in Society: An Introduction to Social Gerontology*, 2nd edition. London: Sage, 304-332.

Hockey J and James A (1993) *Growing Up and Growing Old: Ageing and Dependency in the Life Course*. London: Sage.

Keady J and Nolan MR (1994) Younger-onset dementia: developing a longitudinal model as the basis for a research agenda and as a guide to interventions with sufferers and carers. *Journal of Advanced Nursing* 19, 659-669.

Kitwood T (1993) Person and process in dementia. *International Journal of Geriatric Psychiatry* 8 (7) 541-546.

Newens AJ, Forster DP and Kay DW (1995) Dependency and community care in pre-senile Alzheimer's disease. *British Journal of Psychiatry* 166, 777-782.

O'Brien J, Pearpoint J and Forrest M (1993) *PATH: Planning Alternative Tomorrows with Hope – A Workbook for Planning Possible Positive Futures.* Inclusion Press

Quinn C (1996) *The Care Must Be There: Improving Services for People with Young Onset Dementia and Their Families.* London: The Dementia Relief Trust.

Robertson S (1996) *Younger People with Dementia – the Impact on their Children.* Stirling: Dementia Services Development Centre.

Sperlinger D and Furst M (1994) The service experiences of people with pre-senile dementia: a study of carers in one London borough. *International Journal of Geriatric Psychiatry* 9, 47-50.

Williams O, Keady J and Nolan MR (1995) Younger-onset Alzheimer's disease: learning from the experience of one spouse carer. *Journal of Clinical Nursing* 4(1), 31-36.

Yale R (1995) *Developing Support Groups for Individuals with Early-Stage Alzheimer's Disease.* Baltimore, USA: Health Professions Press.

Wilson SA, Kovach CR and Stearns SA (1996) Hospice concepts in the care for end-stage dementia. *Geriatric Nursing* 17, 6-10.

42 HIV related dementia: the benefits of a small homely environment with a holistic client-centred approach

Buz de Villiers

In the mid-1980s an already embattled community of people trying to cope with the devastating illnesses and social problems caused by HIV disease were confronted by yet another new and frightening issue. AIDS dementia, for many a 'worst nightmare' and at that time an illness of uncertain nature and unknown proportions, was clearly here to stay, bringing with it a host of significant health and social care problems. It has emerged only more recently that it is likely to affect no more than 10 to 15 per cent of all people with AIDS, and that the majority of these will be affected only mildly.

When someone has HIV Related Brain Impairment (HRBI, a wider and more accurate term than dementia) there are two distinct though related care issues:

- the physical problems arising out of the person's HIV disease, which require medical attention primarily, and additionally,
- the fact that there is a fluctuating state of mental impairment, which requires supervision primarily.

In the late 1980s and early 1990s people with moderate/severe HRBI usually ended up being inappropriately 'accommodated' on the wards of the specialist acute care centres, residential care establishments and hospices which provide acute nursing and medical care for people with HIV, simply because there was nowhere else for them to go.

In response to this need, Patrick House was set up to provide care for people with HRBI whose primary need at the time of referral is not for acute nursing or medical care. It is Europe's first, and sadly still its only, residential care service specifically for people with HRBI. Located in west London, Patrick House opened in 1992 and provides accommodation to five people who are so severely affected that they are no longer able to live without constant supervision and support. Twenty-four hour waking cover is provided and the primary form of care on offer is supervision, namely to enable residents to manage the effects of their impairment as independently as possible. However, the aim is to meet all needs as they arise and the project functions as a full nursing home and hospice when required, thereby enabling residents to make it their permanent and last home. The average length of stay is three to six months but this can vary enormously with some clients living at Patrick House for over eighteen months.

When Patrick House was being set up it was thought that the best it would be able to offer would be more appropriate care in a more appropriate setting, but that the individual's mental condition would at best remain static while their physical condition inevitably declined. After more than four years practice with thirty-one residents there have been some very interesting results. While the quality of life of most clients to date has significantly improved, in the case of 35 per cent of residents, particularly those presenting with manic syndromes, there has been a very significant, even dramatic reduction in the behavioural manifestation of their impairment, which has usually been permanent. Some examples of this are given later in this chapter.

What lies behind this unexpected though welcome success? A host of factors play an important part, including the skilled interventions of a well trained, carefully selected, closely supervised and highly motivated care team, as well as the input by externally based professionals from a wide range of multidisciplinary skills, most notably for psychiatric support. However, two features which are unique to Patrick House must take a large share of the credit, namely, the environment and the philosophy and model of care on offer.

The physical environment is comprised of an ordinary but spacious family style home which has been converted and furnished to a very high standard. Residents have the privacy of large double bedrooms with en-suite facilities, overnight guests can be accommodated, and there is ample communal space: a sitting room and large kitchen with attached conservatory that leads onto a garden. The emphasis is on 'ordinariness'. In the bedrooms and the main areas of the house there are few visible signs of design features for disability or safety for example. 'Institutional' aspects, such as the internal lift, mobility bathroom, laundryroom and small staff office have been cleverly designed to be out of the immediate eye. On approaching and entering the building the overwhelming effect is one of 'an ordinary house in an ordinary street' as if one were entering a private home. Residents incur the same levels of risk that they would in their own homes in places like the kitchen, bathroom, stairs and with unlocked doors, for example. The aim is not to eliminate risk altogether but to 'manage' it through close supervision by the care team as appropriate to each individual's capabilities.

Aspects of the philosophy of care ensure that the social and emotional environment is one of a safe, loving, supportive home, and every attempt is made to make the environment as uninstitutional as possible. For example, there are only a minimum number of common sense house rules essential to any shared home, and certainly no rules about getting up, going to bed, going out or meal times. Staff do not wear uniforms or name badges and doors are not marked or locked. Most significantly, a core tenet of the philosophy is that all staff are visitors in the home of the residents, in the same way as the visiting GP for example.

Patrick House has developed its own model of care which is based upon the principles enshrined in the philosophy of care. These principles place great emphasis upon a holistic client-centred approach, and matters such as individualised care planning and delivery, flexibility to meet changing needs, independent living, privacy and dignity, maximisation of quality of life and client advocacy are all regarded as extremely important. The written philosophy is not just a bit of paper filed away. It is a living document to which all staff are continuously encouraged to refer to in their decision making. In practice, staff have needed little encouragement to take ownership of the philosophy, probably because of its common sense, albeit highly idealistic, attempt to enshrine 'best possible practice'.

The resulting model of care is one in which care is delivered by a staff team of trained nurses who do not live-in and provide twenty-four hour waking cover on a 2:5 staff to resident ratio. A strong holistic approach is used so that full cognizance is given to the social, emotional and spiritual aspects of care, in addition to the residents' physical and mental care needs. Complimentary medicine and alternative therapies are encouraged where appropriate, and when the care team themselves cannot deliver these skills, access is made to external sources.

In practice, the client-centred approach means that residents are always consulted in all decision making about their care and the way their home is run, from the big issues such as whether to stop active treatment (of an opportunistic infection), right down to the most trivial matters of daily living. Residents are always encouraged to keep control of their lives, including difficult matters such as their psychotropic medication, and the care team takes every effort to ensure they have a voice, even when they can no longer physically speak. All residents have a personal advocate, usually a partner, best friend or member of the family, who has a formal role in decision making, which is particularly important when the client is severely impaired or receiving terminal care. In this way great effort is taken to ensure that care is never delivered in a manner which is against the wishes of the client.

The model of care is neither formalistic nor prescriptive. The emphasis on flexibility is paramount in delivery of care. Care plans, which are reviewed three times per day, are very detailed and adaptable to changing need or circumstances. The individualised approach means that the subject matter of each resident's care plans could vary enormously, dependent upon individual circumstances.

Another important feature of the model of care is the strongly behavioural approach taken to cognitive impairment issues. While the care of each individual is informed as much as possible by use of brain scans, psychometric testing and the like, these medical assessments are regarded as being of limited value only. The focus of the care approach is on the behavioural manifestation of the individual's cognitive impairment. This includes maintaining a high awareness of the corresponding behaviour of all professional and personal carers involved with the individual as well. Reality orientation is used at all times and inappropriate behaviour is challenged and more positive alternatives are encouraged.

Some examples of how the combination of the environment and the philosophy and model of care have benefited residents, particularly those presenting with manic syndromes, follow:

- *Resident 1* – Presents with severe mania including strong delusions of grandeur and hyperactivity which the hospital ward from which he is referred finds disruptive to the point of further stay being unviable. Within hours of his arrival his main personal carer, a close sibling, visits and finds the degree of improvement remarkable. Within weeks his delusions have disappeared altogether, his hyperactivity continues to decrease to the point that his energy and personality are now a positive asset to the home environment, and his psychotropic medication has been reduced significantly. His energy levels and demands for independence require negotiated risk taking, which includes a fall down the stairs with severe facial bruising as a result, but everyone, including his personal advocate and close family members, agree that his overall quality of life would be poorer if he were more restricted. His insistence on returning home to Ireland for a last visit before dying is not treated as a deluded hope, and is finally realised. He accepts assistance to the airport but otherwise travels independently. In a final case conference he talks with great insight about his period of non-lucidity. He dies peacefully three months after admission to Patrick House and even the quality of his dying is such that he is able to exercise the 'choice' to die just prior to what he terms as 'the hordes descending'.

- *Resident 2* – On admission his personal and professional carers are exasperated, having tried a variety of institutional and home care options. This 'merry-go-round' of care has seemingly done little to alleviate his worsening situation. He is hyperactive, has elevated moods and is generally out of touch with reality. His behaviour is frequently bizarre, for example, preaching from the top of the garden shed and singing hymns in the nearby subway. Within ten weeks he no longer requires any anti-psychotic medication and his behaviour appears to be entirely normal. He lives a full and independent life at Patrick House for eighteen months, including holidays and frequent short visits away. Attempts to move out are considered but fail. At his funeral tribute is paid by those who knew him well to his quality of life and personal growth, including spiritual development, at Patrick House.

- *Resident 3* – Prior to admission he becomes very talkative, disinhibited, hyperactive and grandiose. By the time he is admitted he presents as psychotic with visual hallucinations and is suspicious, frightened and very distressed. He is unable to walk or talk but crawls on the floor 'making noises' in an attempt to communicate. He is doubly incontinent and requires assistance with all personal hygiene. After a period his speech returns permanently and he is able to walk again, though he often has to use a wheelchair. Although he continues to have episodes of hypomania and hallucinations for the rest of his life, these are only periods and much reduced in effect. His psychotropic medication is significantly reduced. His engaging personality and gregarious nature flourish once more. For most of his sixteen month stay at Patrick House he is either at home 'holding court' or out in the local area shopping, at the pub or the cinema. He fulfils his dream of a final holiday abroad in the sun, with the support of friends and the care team.

Finally, a word about the most important factor of all. The overriding message conveyed by the environment and the philosophy and model of care is that of love. Every good carer knows the importance of love, yet its value is often overlooked. This seems to be reflected with our client group, who, in their state of impairment and vulnerability, more than ever simply seem to need to be treated with loving acceptance, which may be something they have not had much experience of before. How difficult it can be for them to ask for it from relative strangers, let alone expect or trust that it will be forthcoming when, for example, their behaviour may be outwardly aggressive or violent. And how challenging for a staff team, themselves simply a group of individuals with a mixed experience of love, to remain connected to warm, open hearted love in the face of extreme physical and emotional distress.

Yet over and again it seems clear that this is what each new client at Patrick House most responds to. In the period of relationship building between client and care team, the unspoken question that always seems to be being tested is something along the lines of: Will you love me, will you always accept me, even though I come across as 'mad' or 'bad' at times because I no longer have full control of my brain's functioning? Will you always be there for me, right through the very very worst, till my death which I know is coming? And when the care team demonstrate that the answer is 'Yes' or 'Mostly, yes' or even 'We'll try our best', the results can be astounding. It is our experience that love is the single most significant factor that underpins our success at Patrick House.

The media

43 Alzheimer in Ballarat

Tom Arie

When I started in old age psychiatry, no one had heard of it except those who worked with mentally ill old people, and silently suffering carers at home. That was in the 1960s. Alzheimer's disease was then known chiefly to medical students, as a rare 'pre-senile' dementia.

Alzheimer's name is now given to the most common of the dementing illnesses, regardless of the age at which it begins, and 'his' disease is a household word, for in one way or another it probably touches most families. The wonderfully successful Alzheimer Societies have spread throughout the world, and are nearly as well known as the Red Cross. There can be few if any universities now in countries like our own that do not have several research projects on the dementias, and this book should give some taste of the nature and range of this great tide of research; and it is hardly possible nowadays to scan a newspaper, or the wireless or television, without encountering the name of Alzheimer. Opening one's paper at breakfast at home, or in Hong Kong or Jerusalem or Toronto or Wanganui one is quite likely to see a headline on dementia or some related topic.

So it is worth recalling one of those little moments when I realised that our cause had become public – that it had 'arrived'.

It was on one of several happy visits to Australia, in the later 1980s. Arthur Harrison, the Melbourne psychiatrist, and his wife Barb, old friends, had taken me on a weekend trip to the one time gold mining town of Ballarat. In a little bookshop there I spotted a Puffin book, *Wilfrid Gordon McDonald Partridge* by Mem Fox.[1] I had heard about it, so I bought a copy.

It is about a small boy and an old lady. They are friends because they have in common that they each have four names. He calls her Miss Nancy (and if you want to know what her other names are, you will have to read the book). People tell him she has lost her memory, but he's not sure what a memory is.

Eventually he finds for her some old and beloved objects, and so helps her to remember – to find her lost memories.

We sat down in a café in the Ballarat Picture Gallery, and the waitress, a girl of about twenty, came to take our order. Beside me on the table she spotted the Puffin book. As she was moving off to get our coffee and cakes, she hesitated, and came back. She looked me confidently in the eye and said, 'I bet you don't know what that book is *really* about. It's about Alzheimer's disease, and you ought to *know* about that. It's *important*.'

And so I ought. And yes, it is. And *she* knew about it. And now almost everyone knows about it. And there's a lot to know.

Note

Wilfrid Gordon McDonald Partridge by Mem Fox, illustrated by Julie Vivas. Picture Puffin. Penguin Books, Harmondsworth, 1987. ISBN 0140505865.

44 Cinderella's rag: refreshing the parts other journals cannnot reach

Sue Benson

My reply to the standard social inquiry 'What do you do?' usually proves a conversation-stopper. The reaction to the news that I edit a journal about dementia is either giggles (rare) or a solemn, anxious expression, 'What a depressing subject that must be'. In all cases it is uphill work to communicate to them that editing a journal on this subject is not all doom and gloom but an area full of new ideas, creativity, progress, warmth, positive thinking and wonderful human beings making it all happen.

But I hardly ever feel I've got any of this across. To my partner in conversation dementia is something they just haven't thought about, and don't want to (even though, increasingly, they are likely to know someone who is affected). It raises anxieties within us all; our defences against that anxiety are strong. Those not in daily contact with dementia can shut it out completely. Even those who *are* in daily contact can shut it out with the 'them and us' attitude which says people with dementia are different, not the same as us, not fully human any more. This 'old culture' of care is very resistant to change, but change is happening nevertheless.

The *Journal of Dementia Care* was born as a reflection of that change and has become an important vehicle for the advance of the 'new culture', which sees the person first and the degenerative disease second, and which knows that effective communication and person-centred care are powerful 'treatments' already available to increase wellbeing.

The Journal is unique in Britain, and perhaps the English-speaking world, in concentrating on care practice (without ignoring the advances of medicine and science). It is written for and by those who work directly with people with dementia, to communicate their thoughts, opinions and discoveries, based on research and experience, about how high quality care and services can be achieved.

It has been welcomed avidly by professional care staff (and many carers too). I believe this is not just because of the opportunity it gives them for education and networking, reading articles written by experts and contributing to it themselves, but above all, the fact that there is a professionally produced journal just for them raises the status of their work. Traditionally the Cinderella of health and social care services, the Journal reveals dementia care (I hope, because this is what I feel) as a fascinating field, both art and science, where the personal qualities of staff, their creativity and inspiration as well as their knowledge and professional skills can be brought into play to achieve small steps and sometimes huge leaps of progress.

So please keep in touch with me at the Journal of Dementia Care, Hawker Publications, 13 Park House, 140 Battersea Park Road. London sw11 4NB. Telephone 0171 720 2108.

Evaluation and critique

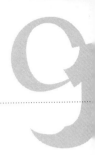

45 Evaluating dementia services

Murna Downs

The purpose of this chapter is to present a brief overview of dementia services' evaluation research. The first part of the chapter describes the limitations of existing services' evaluation research. The second part of the chapter suggests outcomes which may help broaden the focus of future evaluations.

Evaluations concerned with the effect of services have focused almost exclusively on family carers. These studies have produced ambiguous results which have more to do with their methodological difficulties than with any failure of efficacy of the service (for example Levin et al, 1994; Mittelman and Gallagher-Thompson, 1996; Zarit and Teri, 1991). There are at least five methodological weaknesses in these studies which are discussed more fully below.

The service being evaluated may not have been targeted at those carers with the greatest need
It is not always clear that the carers included in the studies had the greatest need for the service. Zarit and Teri (1991) stress the importance of targeting interventions to high-risk groups in order to assess their effectiveness.

Service effects may be diluted due to heterogeneous samples of carers
It is well known that the carers' relation to the person cared for (Colerick and George, 1986; Gilleard, 1984), the quality of their relationship prior to the onset of dementia (Gilhooly, 1986), and whether or not they are living with the person with dementia affect a carer's stress level and coping ability. In addition, Levin et al (1994) suggest that carers differ with respect to their intention to continue caring. As such, these groups may respond differently to interventions. Equally important, there have been several anecdotal reports of the crucial role of timing in ensuring effectiveness of interventions. However, apart from a study by O'Connor et al (1991), the timing of the intervention in

either the course of the dementing illness or in the course of the caring relationship has not been included as an explanatory variable.

Services may not have been provided in sufficient amounts or with carers' needs in mind

The services assessed are often not provided in sufficient amounts and are not always designed with the carer's needs in mind. The notion of a therapeutic dose is well-established in medical research. Nevertheless, social service interventions are frequently assessed at sub-optimal levels. For example, in Lawton et al (1989), the treatment group may not have received a sufficient amount of respite to make a difference. Clearly, researchers have an obligation to include the amount of service use in any equation assessing effectiveness. The relevance for carers of the community-based interventions assessed has been questioned (Gilhooly et al, 1994). Along with Levin et al (1994), they note that carers' need for help at nights and weekend support is rarely addressed by community-based services. Studies which conclude that community-based services are ineffective in supporting carers need to ensure that the services assessed are relevant to their needs.

Outcomes measured may not reflect the aim of the service

The outcomes measured do not always reflect the aims of the service. For example, it has been argued that support groups, which provide opportunities for an exchange of information about dementia and strategies for coping, would be better assessed by examining participants' knowledge and coping rather than their wellbeing or mood. Support groups may have no effect on carers' mood but may be effective in helping carers cope with difficult situations.

Comparisons may be made between groups receiving similar services

Evaluations which employ quasi-experimental designs have difficulty ensuring that the control group receives no treatment (for example Lawton et al, 1989). Carers are not passive, and if they are not included in an experimental intervention they commonly pursue other kinds of support (Zarit and Teri, 1991). As such, it is not uncommon for the experimental and control group to be similar in terms of their service use!

Evaluations which do focus on the effect of services on the person with dementia focus almost exclusively on their likelihood of entering longstay care. It has been argued that this is an inappropriate measure of the effectiveness of community-based services (Ramsay et al, 1995; Zarit, 1990 a,b). The need for alternative measures in assessing the effect of community-based services on people with dementia has been stressed (Ramsay et al, 1995). In particular, the importance of including the perspective of the person with dementia has been stressed (Cotrell and Schulz, 1993).

Outcomes in dementia services' evaluation

Outcomes should reflect the aims of the service. The following list represents examples which might be considered. This list is not intended to be exhaustive. Existing measures of some of these areas have been discussed elsewhere (eg Bowling, 1991, 1995; Kane and Kane, 1981; Lawton and Teresi, 1994; Ramsay et al, 1995; Wilkin and Thompson, 1989).

For people with dementia

- activities of daily living;
- quality of life;
- cognitive functioning;
- depression;
- behaviour problems;
- psychotropic drug use;
- satisfaction with services;
- social activities;
- engagement in activities.

For family carers

- carer stress or burden;
- carer coping ability;
- knowledge about dementia, its prognosis and management;
- physical health (objective and subjective ratings);
- mental health (objective and subjective ratings);
- life satisfaction;
- satisfaction with services.

For formal carers

- communication skills;
- job satisfaction;
- adequacy of leadership;
- quality of care.

There is a clear need for the evaluation and monitoring of dementia services to:

- move beyond service description;
- assess the effect of services on people with dementia and their formal and informal carers; and
- include a variety of outcome measures which reflect the aims of the service as expressed by various stakeholders including people with dementia.

References

Bowling A (1995) *Measuring Disease: A Review of Disease-specific Quality of Life Measurement Scales*. Buckingham: Open University Press.

Bowling A (1991) *Measuring Health: A Review of Quality of Life Measurement Scales*. Buckingham: Open University Press.

Colerick EJ and George LK (1986) Predictors of institutionalisation among caregivers of patients with Alzheimer's disease. *Journal of the American Geriatrics Society* 34, 493-498.

Cotrell V and Schulz R (1993) The perspective of the patient with Alzheimer's Disease: a neglected dimension of dementia research. *Gerontologist* 33, 205-211.

Gilhooly MLM (1986). Senile dementia: factors associated with caregivers' preference for institutional care. *British Journal of Medical Psychology* 56, 165-171.

Gilhooly MLM, Sweeting HN, Whittick JE and McKee K (1994). Family care of the dementing elderly. *International Review of Psychiatry* 6, 29-40.

Gilleard CJ (1984) *Living with Dementia*. London: Croom Helm.

Kane RA and Kane RL (1981) *Assessing the Elderly: a Practical Guide to Measurement*. Lexington, MA: Lexington Books.

Lawton MP, Brody E and Saperstein AR (1989) A controlled study of respite services for caregivers of Alzheimer's patients. *Gerontologist* 29, 8-16.

Lawton MP and Teresi JA (1994) Assessment techniques. *Annual Review of Gerontology and Geriatrics*. 14.

Levin E Moriarty J and Gorbach P (1994. *Better for the Break*. London: HMSO.

Mittelman MS and Gallagher-Thompson D (1996) Valuing intervention research. Letter to the editor. *Journal of Gerontology: Social Sciences* 51B, S268.

O'Connor DW, Pollitt PA, Brook CPB, Reiss BB and Roth M (1991) Does early intervention reduce the number of elderly people with dementia admitted to institutions for long-term care? *British Medical Journal* 302, 871-875.

Ramsay M, Winget C and Higginson I (1995) Review: measures to determine the outcome of community services for people with dementia. *Age and Ageing* 24, 73-83.

Wilkin D and Thompson C (1989) *Users' Guide to Dependency Measures for Elderly People*. Sheffield: Joint Unit for Social Services Research.

Zarit SH (1990a). Issues and directions in family intervention research. In Light E and Lebowitz BD (eds) *Alzheimer's Disease: Treatment and Family Stress*. New York: Hemisphere, 458-486.

Zarit SH (1990b) Interventions with frail elders and their families: are they effective and why? In Stephens MAP, Crowther JH, Hobfoll SE and Tennenbaum DL (eds) *Stress and Coping in Later Life Families*. Washington DC: Hemisphere, 241-262.

Zarit SH and Teri L (1991) Interventions and services for family caregivers. *Annual Review of Gerontology and Geriatrics* 11, 287-310.

Acknowledgements

The author wishes to acknowledge the helpful comments provided by Kate Foster and
Charlie Murphy. Portions of this chapter are based on a Literature Review prepared by the
author for the Northern Ireland Dementia Policy Scrutiny.

46 The continuing quest for predictors of breakdown of family care of elderly people with dementia

Pauline Lightbody and Mary Gilhooly

Despite a proliferation of research over the past two decades, the factors
implicated in the breakdown of family care of elderly people with dementia
remain elusive. In this chapter we begin with an overview of a number of
studies that have been carried out in Britain since the early 1980s, paying
particular attention to informal carers' experience of stress. Following this we
focus on the impact of formal and informal assistance to carers with reference
to the introduction of the Community Care Act. Finally, explanations for the
lack of success in identifying the predictors of breakdown in family care are
highlighted.

The stressful nature of family care

An expanding elderly population has coincided with a shift in emphasis away
from hospital care towards community based provision. However, being cared
for in the community does not mean that the community at large is involved
in providing care; most care received by elderly people comes from their own
families rather than the public sector (Qureshi and Walker, 1986).

Studies involving carers of elderly people with dementia have shown that
between 33 and 75 per cent of carers exceeded the General Health Questionnaire threshold for 'caseness' (that is scores indicating significant emotional
distress) compared to the general population norm of 15 to 20 per cent
(Gilleard et al, 1984; Whittick, 1988). A number of studies also suggest that
caring for mentally impaired elders is more stressful than caring for those
who are physically disabled (Morris et al, 1988). If caring for a relative with
dementia poses special problems, it is vital that the circumstances which
prompt carers to seek institutional care be clearly understood so that
interventions can be correctly targeted.

Predictors of the breakdown of family care

Duration and severity of dementia

Surprisingly, level of severity of the dementia has not often been found to be directly related to caregiver wellbeing. Nevertheless, certain behaviours have been found to be more distressing to carers than others. Because the symptoms of dementia are so varied it can be difficult to isolate aspects which are particularly problematic to caregivers. Behaviours can be categorised as acts of 'omission', for example the inability to prepare a meal or bathe, and acts of 'commission', which include such behaviour as urinating in cupboards and wandering. Acts of commission have been found to be more problematic for caregivers (Gilhooly et al, 1994).

The relationship between duration of illness and carer wellbeing remains unclear; it might be U-shaped rather than a linear function due to the general course of the illness (Orbell and Gillies, 1993). Early symptoms, although less severe, may be more stressful due to uncertainty as to the cause and the changing relationship between the carer and cared-for, whereas advanced cases may enter a more passive state requiring less vigilant attention. This would help to account for the lack of significant findings in correlational studies. Furthermore, although measures of stress taken at initial and follow-up interviews are of interest, they give no indication of how the carers and their dependent relatives fared at the crisis points in between.

Carer characteristics

Current findings indicate that why, and how, care responsibility was assumed, and what, if any, planning preceded the take-over are important factors in predicting current levels of caregiver burden (Karasik, 1995). Responsibility may fall to only one member of the family, which often engenders considerable resentment (Gilhooly, 1987).

Both gender and kinship have been found to affect who takes on a caring role, and there is evidence of an expectation that younger females will care for the frail elderly. Research has consistently shown that men and women experience caring in different ways, with female carers experiencing higher levels of strain than males. Age is also a predictor of burden, with younger carers experiencing greater burden (Kramer and Kipnis, 1995).

Gender differences in the provision of care are less marked in older age groups as care is increasingly encapsulated within marriage. Spouse carers account for approximately one third of all informal care (Arber and Ginn, 1991) and have been found to be less likely to seek institutional care (Collerick and George, 1986). However spouse carers are usually also co-resident which is another factor found to predict continued caregiving. The quality of the pre-morbid relationship has been found to impinge on the caring situation

(Gilleard, 1985; Gilhooly, 1986) and it is often assumed that a long and happy marriage will motivate a husband or wife to provide care. However, there seems to be little basis for assuming that a long relationship will necessarily have been a happy one. Perhaps not all old and frail people 'deserve to be cared for by their families'!

The impact of formal and informal assistance to carers
Social support has been found to moderate the effects of caregiver stress (Gallo, 1990). However, the relationship between the amount of help received by carers and stress is unclear. Research has shown that it is not the amount of assistance given that matters, but rather satisfaction with the assistance (Wethington and Kessler, 1986).

In general the provision of services has not been found to be related to reduced levels of stress, improved wellbeing, or lower rates of institutionalisation (Gilhooly, 1990). However, care of elderly people has traditionally tended to slot people into a limited number of available services, few of which have had the explicit aim of supporting informal carers. Many services have been designed to overcome the problems posed by 'acts of omission' whereas it is the 'acts of commission' which are most problematic (Gilhooly, 1994).

Most carers would prefer that their dependent relatives did not enter long term care. However, our own research has shown that even when carers indicate their willingness to continue in their role it does not always prove to be possible. If maintenance of people with dementia within the community becomes a goal in itself, local authorities may find themselves wasting valuable resources targeting services at an insurmountable problem. Community care is not necessarily a cheaper option.

Method and the meaning of research findings

A number of issues have been raised concerning research relating to the family care of elderly people with dementia.

It has been suggested that one of the major problems has been with the methodology employed. Because of the limited number of services available there is insufficient variance in service provision to produce a statistically significant correlation between provision and the outcome measure, irrespective of how important the service was to carers. The independent variables are also often interlinked, for example co-residence often implies either a spouse-carer, or a dependent whose disability is so severe as to prohibit independent living; any effect associated with age may be confounded by the carer/dependant relationship (Wenger, 1990). Montgomery suggests that the confounding of independent variables is such that it is almost impossible to summarise the relationships between caregiver characteristics or burden with any definitive statement (Montgomery, 1991).

In a critique of the caregiving literature, Barer and Johnson (1990) identified such problems as the confused definition of 'caregiver', the diversity of help required and received, the over-representation of self-selected samples, and the lack of acknowledgement of secondary carers The authors claimed that due to methodological faults both researchers and practitioners lacked a clear insight into the caregiving process. Dura and Kiecolt-Glaser (1990) also highlighted problems with sample bias in caregiving research, and point out that recruitment of subjects can significantly affect results. We would also argue that what is needed is more qualitative research, systematic evaluations of interventions, and the inclusion of the dementia sufferers themselves in research studies.

Concluding comments

It was not until the early 1980s that the vast amount of work involved in providing informal care was properly acknowledged. The majority of early, 'first generation' studies aimed to provide a broad overview of the caring situation. It is hoped that the later, 'second generation' studies, which tend to be more tightly focused, will overcome some of the methodological problems identified above. However, a narrow remit may result in findings largely of academic interest, rather than providing the basis for social policy.

The philosophy of community care is committed to maintaining independence in the community. However, it must be acknowledged that caring for someone who is unable to care for themselves or communicate in any meaningful way actually deprives carers of their own independence. Services need to be directed at goals that enhance the meaning of life for both the carer and the cared-for, rather than simply assuring survival and postponing institutionalisation. Future research needs to be geared towards identifying the signs of approaching crisis, not necessarily to increase service provision, but in order to defuse the crisis and ease the transition into care which in many cases is inevitable. Institutionalisation should not be seen as a failure, but as a stage in the process of caring which should be entered into at a point which will cause the least distress to the sufferer and at which carers are still able to pick the threads of their own lives.

References

Arber S and Ginn J (1991) *Gender and Later Life: A Sociological Analysis of Resources and Constraints*. London: Sage.

Barer MB and Johnson CL (1990) A critique of the caregiving literature. *The Gerontologist* 30(1), 26-29.

Collerick EJ and George LK (1986) Predictors of institutionalization among caregivers of patients with Alzheimer's disease. *Journal of the American Geriatrics Society* 34, 493-498.

Dura JR and Kiecolt-Glaser JK (1990). Sample bias in caregiving research. *Journal of Gerontology: Psychological Sciences* 45(5), 200-204.

Gallo J (1990) The effect of social support on depression in caregivers of the elderly. *The Journal of Family Practice* 30, 430-440.

Gilhooly MLM (1986) Senile dementia: factors associated with care-givers' preference for institutional care. *British Journal of Medical Psychology* 56, 165-171.

Gilhooly MLM (1987) Dementia and the family. In Orford J (ed) *Coping with Disorder in the Family*. London: Croom Helm.

Gilhooly MLM (1990) Do Services Prevent or Delay Institutionalisation of People with Dementia? Research Report 4. Stirling: Dementia Services Development Centre.

Gilhooly MLM (1994) The social dimensions of senile dementia. In Hanley I and Hodge J (eds) *Psychological Approaches to the Care of the Elderly*. London: Croom Helm, 88-135.

Gilhooly MLM, Sweeting HN, Whittick JE and McKee K (1994) Family care of the dementing elderly. *International Review of Psychiatry* 6, 29-40.

Gilleard CJ (1985) Predicting the outcome of psychogeriatric day care. *The Gerontologist* 25, 280-285.

Gilleard CJ et al (1984) Emotional distress amongst the supporters of the elderly mentally infirm. *British Journal of Psychiatry* 145, 172-177.

Karasik RJ (1995) Becoming a caregiver: siblings assuming care roles for older aduls with development disabilities. Paper presented at the 48th annual meeting of the Gerontological Society of America. Abstract published in *The Gerontologist* 31(1), 123.

Kramer BJ and Kipnis S (1995) Eldercare and work-role conflict: toward an understanding of gender differences in caregiver burden. *The Gerontologist* 35(3), 340-348.

Montgomery RJV (1991) Investigating caregiver burden. In Markides KS and Cooper CL (eds) *Ageing, Stress and Health*. Essex: Wiley.

Morris LW, Morris RG and Birtton PG (1988) The relationship between marital intimacy, perceived strain and depression in spouse care-givers of dementia sufferers. *British Journal of Medical Psychology* 62, 173-179.

Orbell S and Gillies B (1993) What's stressful about caregiving? *Journal of Applied Social Psychology* 23(4), 272-290.

Qureshi H and Walker A (1986) Caring for elderly people: the family and the state. In Phillipson C and Walker A (eds) *Ageing and Social Policy: a Critical Assessment*. Aldershot: Gower.

Ray M (1995) Spouse care in the context of long term marriage relationships. *Generations Review* 5(2), 6-8.

Wenger C (1990) Change and adaptation in informal support networks of elderly people in Wales 1979-87. *Journal of Aging Studies* 4(4), 375-389.

Wethington E and Kessler RC (1986) Perceived support, received support and adjustment to stressful life events. *Journal of Health and Social Behaviour* 27, 78-89.

Whittick K (1988) Dementia and mental handicap: attitudes and emotional distress in carers. *British Journal of Clinical Psychology* 27, 167-172.

Sex, death and spirituality

47 Sexuality and dementia?

Carole Archibald

In this, the latter part of the twentieth century, sex and sexual images abound. 'We live, in short, in a sexualised world' (Hawkes, 1996 p1). Films, in terms of sexuality, start where they once finished. Gay sexuality is celebrated on film and in written work and many venues. Practices such as sado-masochism, the use of sex toys, and issues such as every woman's right to multiple orgasms are regularly aired in magazines. Yet these sexual images are partial. They are essentially of youth: lithe young bodies, beautiful and sexually assertive. The world has an increasing store of what Plummer (1995) refers to as 'sexual stories'. However these tend not to be the sexual stories of older people or people with dementia.

What is interesting to ponder is whether or not this will change. Will the young people of today have sexual stories to tell when they are old? How will they address their sexual needs as they become old and possibly demented or if they are admitted into residential care? Will they conform to society's stereotypical, often asexual, view of old people or will they continue to assert their interest? Will those that retain an interest, and are still sexually active, take their 'equipment' into the residential home and/or continue their relationships? If they are gay or lesbian will they be able to acknowledge their relationships or will they remain closeted? Barbara McDonald (1984) in a thought provoking book on her life and her experience as a lesbian asks what has happened to all the young lesbians she had affairs with in the 1960s. Where are they now? In the year 2020 will there have been a sea change in attitudes and ideas?

As we approach the millennium and beyond, the state of the art in dementia care is towards a recognition and acknowledgement of the person with dementia while also being aware of the needs of the carer. In the not too distant past all effort was made to address the needs of the carer. There was often scant recognition of the psychological needs of the person with dementia.

Now there is an increasing awareness that dementia although an insidious and a dreadful disease, is just that. It is a disability visited on the person. The person, as an adult person, remains there throughout. Good practice is increasingly being associated with what is referred to as 'person centred care' (Kitwood and Bredin, 1992). This is care which has, at the focus, the person with dementia and their needs. It is an approach in which the wellbeing of the person is uppermost. It is an exemplary approach but it is an approach which requires some scrutiny and exploration in the context of sexuality and people with dementia.

It is generally accepted that sexual expression not only involves the 'person' but can, and often does, involve others, whose needs also have to be considered. This is particularly so in dementia. For example, what happens if the person with dementia needs and demands sexual intimacy which the carer is no longer able to provide? Reciprocity, an important aspect of any relationship, can be missing in dementia. Roles may change as the carer takes on increasing responsibilities. The carer may no longer view that person as a sexual partner. They may feel distaste or see any intimacy almost as akin to incest. Which person's needs are paramount? What happens if the person with dementia is admitted to residential care and expresses sexual need towards staff or other residents or masturbates in public? Training materials (Archibald, 1994) and the provision of workshops are starting to address how staff might work through some of these situations. The bottom line however remains: if the person with dementia expresses a need for a sexual relationship with another person, and a partner is not available, this need cannot be met. Staff cannot procure and it is questionable whether the idea of sex toys as a means of addressing need has been considered. In one nursing home in Australia, erotic videos and magazines were made available to certain male residents as a means of addressing their sexual needs, but this tends not to be common practice.

These kinds of issues need to be considered. They need to be considered not least because of the legal implications and the duty to care, but importantly by considering them, a reframing of the situation results. In this reframing, there is a recognition that the person with dementia is an adult being with adult status and possibly sexual needs. Adult status, which includes the acceptance of a person as a sexual being, is symbolised by autonomy, self-determination and choice (Hockey and James, 1993). The concept of personhood prevails, with its attendant full membership of society. These factors, central to the philosophy of person centred care, are often missing in the life of someone with dementia. But adult status also confers responsibilty; responsibility for one's own actions which can be missing as the disease progresses. Being adult would also suggest that there is a consideration taken of other people's needs. Being self-centred and irresponsible is not always the result of dementia. People who do not have dementia can be self-centred and irresponsible but these aspects of personality can be accentuated in some people as the disease progresses, and this can impact on sexual expression.

There is a dearth of studies on sexuality and dementia. Kellett (1989) notes anecdotally, 'that men who continue to make love to their demented wives generally remain more effective carers'. This acknowledges some of the positives. Most of the studies tend to portray sexuality and dementia as problematic (Zeisss et al, 1990; Nadal and Allgulander, 1993; Haddad, 1993 a, b; Alexopoulos, 1994). The literature on carers of people with dementia and sexuality can also tend towards the problematic (Brett et al, 1990; Kuhn, 1994). Dementia brings in its train sexual behaviours which can be problematic, if not for the person, problematic for carers and professional carers. These can result in aggression/sexual aggression, and loss of short-term memory so the person can forget that they may have only recently had sex. There may be misrecognition so the person approaches the wrong person in a sexual way. There may be sexual abuse of the person with dementia due to their vulnerability, or the person with dementia may become the abuser.

In some people dementia can result in sexual disinhibition. Where previously a woman may have either had few or no partners, she might actively seek out a partner and obtain pleasure from the encounter. Men or women who perhaps have had latent homosexual leanings but have married and had children, now choose a partner of the same sex. If these scenarios occur in residential care homes for example should the decision be based on the person's past, or their present needs? Should the person be protected from themself and the ravages of the disease or should the relationship continue if they are deriving some pleasure and people's rights are intact? If there is a carer (partner) involved, what of their needs?

Staff also have needs which have to be considered. They bring to the situation their own agendas, feelings, prejudices and past experiences of sexuality. Sexual desire is a basic human drive and need but unfettered there is a sense, for many, of uncontrollability about it (Hawkes, 1996). There is something uncontrollable and unpredictable too about dementia that seems to evoke strong emotions and a desire to protect and control.

Some consider there is a need for constant surveillance. Sexuality and dementia seems to be an issue for staff but this has not been reflected in policies and guidelines (Parkin, 1989).

The problems associated with sexuality and dementia need to be acknowledged and discussed as a starting point. The person centred approach in the area of sexuality and dementia remains problematic (but not insurmountable) if all 'persons' needs are considered. If the person with dementia and their needs can be central and the person included in the discussion, even in the later stages of the disease (Lichtenberg and Strzpek, 1990), then progress will have been made.

The person with dementia, as with everyone, is many faceted. When dementia intervenes they have like all of us a past, a present and an uncertain future. They have a biography that will include relationships of many kinds. These relationships will have affected their lives and some (perhaps recently formed relationships) will remain central to their wellbeing. If care is to be person centred it may be important, and pertinent for some people, that these relationships, including sexual relationships, are explored in a sensitive and discreet way, and affirmed.

Sexuality generally has now come of age (Jackson and Scott, 1996) but the area of sexuality and dementia remains for the most part undisturbed. 'Omission is a powerful statement' according to Starr and Weiner (1981). Perhaps the state of the art in dementia care is learning to address this silence, sensitively and carefully. Giddens (1992) talks of sexual freedom following power and being an expression of that power. Is it possible to give this power, this sexual power to those people with dementia who want it, and if so, 'how'?

References

Alexopulos P (1994) Management of sexually disinhibited behaviour by a dementia patient. *Australian Journal on Ageing* 13(3).

Archibald C (1994) *Sexuality and Dementia: A Guide*. Stirling: Dementia Services Development Centre.

Brett TL, Zeiss MA and Davies H (1990) Sexual concerns of male spouses of female Alzheimer's disease patients. *The Gerontologist* 30(1).

Giddens A (1992) *The Transformation of Intimacy*. London: Polity Press

Haddad P and Benbow S (1993a) Sexual problems associated with dementia: Part 1. Aetiology, assessment and treatment. *International Journal of Geriatric Psychiatry* 8, 631-637.

Haddad P and Benbow S (1993b) Sexual problems associated with dementia: Part 2. Problems and their consequences. *International Journal of Geriatric Psychiatry* 8, 547-551.

Hawkes G (1996) *A Sociology of Sex and Sexuality*. Buckingham: Open University Press.

Hockey J and James A (1993) *Growing Up, Growing Old*. London: Sage.

Jackson S and Scott S (1996) *Sexual Skirmishes and Feminist Factions: Twenty Five Years of Debate on Women and Sexuality*. Forthcoming.

Kellett J (1989) The reality of sexual behaviour in old age: there's a lot of it about. *Geriatric Medicine* October, 17-18.

Kitwood T and Bredin K (1992) Towards a theory of dementia care: personhood and well-being. *Ageing and Society* 12, 269-287.

Kuhn RD (1994) The changing face of sexual intimacy in Alzheimer's disease. *The American Journal of Alzheimer's Care and Related Disorders and Research*, September/October.

Lichtenberg P and Strzpek D (1990) Assessment of institutionalised dementia patients' competencies to participate in intimate relationships. *The Gerontologist* 30(1), 117-120.

McDonald B and Rich C (1984) *Look Me in the Eye*. London: The Women's Press.

Nadal M and Allgulander S (1993) Normalisation of sexual behaviour in a female with dementia after treatment with cyproterone. *International Journal of Geriatric Psychiatry* 8, 265-267.

Parkin W (1989) Private experiences in the public domain: sexuality and residential care organisations. In Hearn J, Sheppard DL, Sherriff-Tancred P and Burrell G (eds) *The Sexuality of Organisations*. London: Sage.

Plummer K (1995) *Telling Sexual Stories*. London: Routledge.

Scott S and Jackson S (1996) Sexual skirmishes and feminist factions: twenty-five years of debate on women and sexuality. In Jackson S and Scott S (eds) *Feminism and Sexuality*. Edinburgh University Press.

Starr BD and Weiner MB (1981) *Report on Sex and Sexuality in the Mature Years*. London: WH Allen.

Zeiss AM, Davis HM, Wood M and Tinklenberg JR (1990) The incidence and correlates of erectile problems in patients with Alzheimer's disease. *Archives of Sexual Behaviour* 19, 325-332.

48 Talking about death

Mary Dixon

Mr and Mrs Mair were referred to the community care team I work in, by their daughter Marjory. Mrs Mair was described as experiencing problems due to her poor short term memory, she could be easily upset by changes to her routine and was sometimes agitated with those around her. Her frail 90 year old husband was struggling to provide the care she needed. However his own health was poor, he suffered from respiratory problems and was quite arthritic. A community care assessment was requested to see what help the social work department might be able to offer. Over the course of a few months I got to know the couple and their family fairly well. I put together a day care package, applied for Attendance Allowance for both and cajoled their GP in to making a referral for a formal diagnosis of Mrs Mair's dementia. The family began to feel comfortable and confident with my intervention. Our contact was very relaxed and I felt they looked forward to my visits. We talked about respite care, planning this for the future and often shared a good humoured joke. All in all I felt the assessment was a good one.

Suddenly, at the turn of the year, Mr Mair became ill and died within three days of admission to hospital. The close knit family were shocked and soon torn apart by their grief. Central to their distress was the reaction of Mrs Mair, to losing her partner of sixty-two years. She had visited him in hospital, been with him when he died, attended his funeral. But all with no reaction, no obvious grief. At the graveside her only action was to nudge her daughter and ask what time they would be going home for dinner.

At first the general assumption made was that her reaction was dictated by her dementia. The family felt that she did not understand what was happening, she did not mention her husband because she did not remember him ever having existed, or, that she had simply forgotten the events of the last week. Her lack of reaction was very hard for them to accept. I also found myself wondering at how cruel it was that her dementia should seem to rob her of the ability to react appropriately to the events around her.

As I came to reflect on my role with the couple I thought about what I knew about Mrs Mair. The truth was, not as much as I had given myself credit for. I had not really managed, as part of my assessment, to talk to Mrs Mair with any true depth. I knew a number of things about her, her major life events, some of her joys and some of her disappointments. But I did not know how she dealt with death. I knew little in any detail about how she had experienced bereavements or how she had come to terms with previous losses in her life. I had listened to her talk about her own parents, but had never asked her how much she missed them. I had not thought to give her time and encouragement to talk about them, to possibly revisit feelings of loss and sadness. I made an assumption that such conversations were about her experiencing her past as her present and that this would be the only reason she might want to talk about her parents.

Mrs Mair stayed on at home after her husband died, but only for a few weeks. She and her family could not cope with her range of care needs and so she moved on to nursing home care. Over the following months the nursing home staff commented that Mrs Mair was occasionally weepy and that once or twice she had asked staff where her husband was. At other times she volunteered the information that he had been in hospital and was now dead.. Throughout this time I talked with her family, and the nursing staff caring for her, about how we could best offer Mrs Mair comfort and support. We recognised that it would help us if we could encourage her to talk about her feelings. But we did not know if this was what she would want to do. We did not know how private a person she might be in terms of talking about her feelings, or if indeed she would chose to talk to us about how she felt.

Mrs Mair had now experienced two massive changes, the loss of her husband and the move to care. This and her impaired memory of recent events left us floundering to know what to do for the best. We did not know if she would have the capacity to think about her feelings or if she could find the words to clearly express what she felt. Would her dementia have taken away all her abilities to experience and give voice to feelings of anger and denial? Would the dementia impact on her ability to eventually come to some reconciliation of her loss?

Finally, we developed a course of action. Mrs Mair's family felt it was too upsetting and unsettling if staff regularly made a point of trying to raise the topic of her husband with her. We agreed we would respond and talk with her, only when she wished to talk about him. We confirmed that we would remind her, if this was needed, that her husband was dead. However our preferred course of action would be to guide her, so that she could remember this information and acknowledge for herself that he was dead. In hindsight I feel that by not taking the initiative and raising the subject with her, she may not have felt able to recognise at times why she felt so troubled.

In looking back now, seven months after her loss I feel I know Mrs Mair a lot better. I see her as someone who was in shock when her husband died. She worried about her children's tears and distress but was unable to reach out and protect them as she felt she should. She could not physically attend to the making of the funeral arrangements so let others step into what should have been her place. The family did not think to encourage her to share in these tasks and she did not ask. Mrs Mair was someone who needed a long time and a lot of gentle concern and care before she could share with others how she felt. Sometimes she looked worried and sad, she knew something was terribly wrong but she could not think what it was. She needed us not to be afraid to broach the subject with her, but to relieve the build-up of tension that she was experiencing, so that she could then remember, cry and miss her husband.

In working with Mrs Mair I started to think about the number of other times I have talked about death with an older person. Several years ago I had to break the news of a death to a 85 year old woman with dementia. She had shared her home and her entire life with her 79 year old sister whom had died suddenly. During the first few hours that I sat with her, Ada asked for her sister Rhona, over and over again. Each time that I had to explain that she was dead, I felt this news was akin to striking her. She would look stunned, burst into tears and sob for ten minutes. When she finally stopped, we would have a cup of tea, she would look at me quite calmly and again ask where Rhona was.

This constant battering exhausted us both. Ada died four months after her sister. I felt then, as I do now, that I had to tell Ada the truth. It would have beeen too difficult to create an excuse not to answer her questions or to try and change the subject. But the toll it took on her was awful to watch.

From talking with colleagues I began to hear that others found themselves grappling with some of the same issues and that their experiences, reactions and stories were certainly as varied as my own. A psychiatrist friend wondered about the intellectual and reasoning abilities a person with dementia would have retained in order to be able to work through a bereavement process. She worried whether someone could get stuck at a particular stage in the process and so be unable to move on to any acceptance of what had happened. A colleague running a home support service talked of a woman she had visited just recently who had lost her daughter. The older woman and her daughter had shared a bedroom for the last six years since the diagnosis of dementia had been made. When the old woman would wake in the night her daughter was there to reach out a reassuring hand to hold onto, until she fell asleep again. When the daughter died, her brothers never mentioned her again to their mother. They hoped she would forget and so spare herself the distress of realising her terrible loss. When she asked where her daughter was, her family told her she was out at the shops. The same worker also knew of a 76 year old woman who had been living with her daughter, son in law and three grandsons. When her daughter died, her family, like the one in the previous example, did not want her distressed and upset. She moved to live with another daughter who could attend to her very personal care needs. However, she talked with the worker about how she liked to visit her former home. Particularly to be with her youngest grandson. She confided to the worker, that he still had the smell of her daughter on him. She could not talk about her daughter to anyone else because her other children could not cope.

I have no answers to suggest as to how we might handle this subject. I see it as a gap I had not thought about until recently. It will be on my agenda from now on as part of all further assessments. Maybe though we do need to start thinking and talking about these experiences to try and find some common way to help those in most distress.

49 Spiritual needs and religious practice in dementia care

Alison Froggatt and Laraine Moffitt

Awareness of the spiritual and religious in the dementia process developed alongside increased understanding in the social and emotional spheres. The process has been similar, collecting clues from observant family and professional carers, and reflecting on them. People attempting to meet the ongoing religious and spiritual needs of their relatives with severe memory loss have made a significant contribution.

Defining spirituality is always tricky. In this context we mean the search for that which gives zest, energy, meaning and identity to a person's life, in relation to all other people, and to the wider world. Spirituality can be experienced in feelings of awe or wonder, those moments of life which take you beyond the mundane into a sacred space. In this chapter we want to focus more specifically on religious ways of meeting spiritual needs

A person's religious needs are more specifically related to faith, history, the framework of beliefs, and the community, institutional and organisational components of a particular church, mosque, temple, synagogue or worship centre. The ritualistic ways in which such a person is reminded to maintain hope and trust in the Almighty are particularly important where there is memory loss. For some people spirituality may be concerned with the experiential side of religion as opposed to the rules and organisational demands. Those who do not hold religious beliefs also have spiritual awareness and needs.

New approaches to dementia include those which focus on the experience of the individual trapped inside a deteriorating mental capacity (Kitwood and Benson, 1995), recognising that the person with dementia continues to have feelings, The spiritual aspect is integral (Froggatt, 1994; Barnett, 1995; Kitwood et al, 1995; Moffitt, 1996). Thus it is that government guidelines for inspectors in residential and nursing homes now expect attention to be paid to spiritual needs. The experience of the chaplaincy project in Newcastle is that residential care homes are wanting to be able to ensure that spiritual needs are being met. Some research has begun to recognise this dimension (Kitwood et al, 1995 p32).

There is a cost to developing one's spiritual and religious awareness in relation to people with dementia. It requires participation in depth from spouse, carer, care assistant or chaplain. Spirit meets spirit as flame touches flame, and sometimes one is burned. Barnett (1995) fluently explores this kind of self-giving awareness in that no one accompanying a dementia journey can do so without feeling pain and some distress. A specific example of this is given in *Holy Holy Holy* (Treetops, 1996). Both the hysterical crying of the patient who called out 'Help me Jesus help me' and the serene peaceful behaviour of another patient, were carried spiritually by the chaplain of the home.

In this area of work much needs to be done to develop understanding of the spiritual and religious needs of carers (family and professionals) as well as those with brain failure both in places of worship, in the community and in residential and nursing care.

Working with spiritual and religious aspects combines celebration, commemoration and compassion. Celebration involves more than active enjoyment and a feeling of pleasure. One kind of celebration might be to visit someone taking flowers, especially ones with a good smell to help trigger off memories of past happiness at a deep level, and lead to a sense of enjoyment and celebration of the Other (Shamy, 1993). On the other hand the rich variety of appropriate religious festivals would be another way of celebrating, as well as community festivals for everyone like Harvest Festival and Christmas.

Commemoration involves ritual, and repetition of familiar phrases. This may be well loved stories or poetry, as well as songs, hymns or prayers, and the use of artifacts such as a rosary or crucifix, for Roman Catholics, a Bible or hymn book for Protestants, a prayer mat for Muslims.

Compassion involves a readiness to enter into the dementing process and see what it must feel like emotionally and spiritually as has been described above (Treetops, 1996 p9). Many can find themselves responding with compassion and love in a way that feeds the vitality and zest of a person. The spiritual and religious aspects are inextricably interwoven with the practical aspects of life for it is in material ways that we can express ourselves most easily.

In order to begin to meet religious needs it is important to take note of a person's faith history, with the help of family and friends if necessary, and write down what has been learned. First find out the religion, and if a Christian, the denomination: Roman Catholic, Church of England, Methodist, Salvationist, Quaker, Pentecostal. It may be that a person was an atheist deliberately not having any religious faith.

Next find out which place of worship was attended, how regularly and how recently. If it is nearby the connections with that group could still be encouraged. Did the person have any particular responsibility? Was he or she a leading figure in the past? Did religious observance matter a lot to the person?

Then one can begin to find the appropriate way to obtain some ritual and symbolism to remind the person of their faith.

In a residential setting it is helpful to most christians present to have a minister or priest come in to bring Holy Communion. The ritual activity of being offered bread and wine reaches many people with dementia and is a reassurance of God's love, as well as that of the church outside the home. Theologically it is also an actual reassurance of the presence of Christ with that person, which is not dependent on the measure of the person's immediate response.

The way in which religious words can reach in is demonstrated by the following incident. An officer in charge of a home was in the habit of saying 'May God remember you and bless you' to each resident as she went round saying goodnight. One woman with dementia who talked incessantly stopped, looked her straight in the eye and said, 'Yes, I will try and remember that'.

Ritual gives a sense of familiarity, and therefore of safety and comfort. It is repetitive, therefore you know what to expect. It acts as a strong memory cue. There are few surprises to provoke confusion. As Buckland found in his research (Kitwood et al, 1995 p33):

> *Being part of a well learned ritual can give respite from feelings of confusion...those who believe in God and continue to have a formal link with God may gain a sense of security through that link.*

There are many stories of people without speech or memory finding the words to continue a prayer that someone else has started. One correspondent told us, 'When I visited my mother in her nursing home, and she was as usual saying how scared she was, I took a deep breath and said "I'll tell you what, let's say 'Our Father' together". She got all the way through with scarcely a hesitation. There was a pause, and then she looked me straight in the eye and said "Thank you darling". It was a real contact and very moving.'

Hymns, as with songs, provide particularly strong memory cues. We observed at a service in a residential home a new resident seemed to have memory loss, and jumbled speech. The first hymn chosen by other residents was *The Lord's my shepherd, I'll not want*. Everyone sang with feeling and he joined in. By the end of the first verse he was weeping, and a sensitive care assistant perched herself on the arm of his chair and found a handkerchief. At the end of the hymn he said clearly, 'That was lovely'.

Even though the memories evoked were sad, he was restored to some sense of who he was and what had mattered to him. Later, as he settled in we realised he was a good singer who much enjoyed familiar hymns.

Keeping someone with severe memory loss connected to their faith community does rely on past memory of habit, of place, of people, the accretions of memories of worship built up in the past. Someone living alone and coping with brain failure may have a clear picture of being a religious person but may be unable to remember to participate. Thus the worshipping community has to hold the faith memory of the person, welcome them lovingly and uncritically. This may involve adjustments to unexpected or even slightly antisocial behaviour. That which is acceptable in a small child restlessness, talking loudly, wandering, even incontinence, may be less acceptable in adults. So work needs to go on in a faith community to appreciate what being loving and accepting involves. One church was able to allow their former treasurer even in quite severe dementia to follow her ritual of counting the money after the service, before going home with her family.

The question of hope in dementia is an important one. Spiritual and religious nurture increases hope, the sense that all is well and will be well. By contrast where a person is treated unkindly or abandoned by family, even a religious person may lose faith in God (Kitwood and Benson, 1995 p70). Religious stimuli may bring back unhappy memories, or the person may feel it one thing more than they can bear to cope with. We have seen someone who had been able to respond to a service in a home reach a place of withdrawal and say 'Go away, I don't want that'. The fact that a person has been in contact momentarily does not mean this capacity will continue as the disease progresses.

Those who can receive religious or spiritual nurture do seem to have an hour or two of greater peace and less restlessness, even if it is not possible to remember the cause of it. And there is every reason to suppose that those from other faiths, at present in the minority in many residential settings, will also benefit from sensitive awareness of their religious as well as cultural customs, and significant rituals. There are many more handbooks available to help staff understand what is needed (Squires, 1991). All the issues to do with help for people from black and minority communities who have dementia have been relatively under-researched (Nearby, 1991). In many faiths dietary observances and times of fasting are as much a part of their religious life as times for prayer and the correct ablutions. We can learn afresh from considering different religions how faith involves the whole of life, and care should be taken with all the important details, particularly in residential homes (Froggatt, 1991).

For carers, too, religious support and spiritual awareness may help to answer some of the difficult questions. Many inner resources are needed to keep a sense of stability and meaning throughout this shadowy time, to remember who the person was, and yet sustain all the uncomfortable daily realities. Where religious needs can be sufficiently met the person receives the sense of belonging and being known and accepted. They know in some sense that they are remembered by God, and have a hope of salvation when present difficulties end. In helping to meet spiritual needs, one is sustaining deeper memory. To lose that is to lose power and to lose wholeness. 'Re-membering: putting together and reconnecting all the fragments and dismembered elements of experience is part of the recovery of a lost sense of wholeness' (Grey, 1989 p10).

Reflecting our own experience this chapter has been biased towards the needs of Christians with dementia, but the principles are relevant for all stages of diverse belief and none.These can only be glimpses of the rich field of understanding faith memory and spiritual awareness in the dementia process; put together all you know of any particular person to find clues and cues that will give some healing of spirit, to recover more wholeness and hope.

References

Barnett E (1995) Broadening our approach to spirituality. In Kitwood T and Benson's (eds) *The New Culture of Dementia Care*. London: Hawker Publications.

Nearby J (1991) *A Hidden Problem? Dementia Amongst Minority Ethnic Groups*. Stirling: Dementia Services Development Centre.

Froggatt A (1991) Inner beliefs. *Community Care* 876, 15-16.

Froggatt A (1994) Tuning in to spiritual needs. *Journal of Dementia* Care 2(2).

Grey M (1989) *Redeeming the Dream*. London: SPCK.

Kitwood T and Bredin K (1992) Towards a theory of dementia care: personhood and well-being. *Ageing and Society* 12, 269-287.

Kitwood T and Benson's (eds) (1995) *The New Culture of Dementia Care*. London: Hawker Publications.

Kitwood T, Buckland's and Petrie T (1995) *Brighter Futures*. Oxford: Anchor Housing.

Moffitt L (1996) Helping to create sacred space. *Journal of Dementia Care* 4(3).

Shamy E (1993) *Spiritual Needs of People with Dementia*. Stirling: Dementia Services Development Centre.

Squires A (ed) (1991) *Multicultural Health Care and Rehabilitation of Older People*. London: Edward Arnold with Age Concern.

Treetops J (1996) *Holy Holy Holy Faith in Elderly People* (Leeds) 53 Cardigan Lane, Leeds LS4 2LE.

50 From factory to hearth: valuing humanness in dementia care

Monica Nebauer and Kim Wylie

The western political doctrine of economic rationalism reflects a market place ideology of privatisation, 'user pays' and effective time management. Despite such political and economic pressures, aged and dementia care has an exciting opportunity of responding to the prevailing shift of reductionism to holism, by rejecting the biomedical or 'disease' approach to care and focusing on the humanistic values inherent in a more holistic approach to care. Consequently, this chapter is about a nursing 'dream' for a humanistic, holistic approach to state of the art in dementia care and will explore some of the present day attitudes, institutional problems and concerns that prevent the realisation of this dream.

The biomedical (disease) focus of care

Dementia is equated with disability and disease, consequently, care for dementing residents is provided under the umbrella of a biomedical model, in which Cartesian dualism snares the human body in the analogy of the German word *Korper*, which means 'physical body'. In this sense, the *Korper* is seen as the 'object body' which is observed from without from a third person perspective, and is simply an example of a classification of a physical thing (Leder, 1990). Imaging the dementing elder in such an objective, mechanistic way results in an emphasis on disembodying, mechanistic and positivist approaches such as chemical and physical restraint which condemn these people to a life of meaningless existence.

In efficient and profitable aged care dementia facilities (referred to by some nurses as factories or labour camps) many nurses rely on devices provided by the technological world such as bodycare, bodymover and bodycontrol tools. Bodycare tools are usually neatly stored in ergonomically safe trolleys along corridor walls. These trolleys are piled high with special sheets to catch and absorb the drips and the solid matter excreted by the tonne each day. There are also rags for cleaning bottoms, plastic drainage bags to hook onto tubes that poke out of bottoms and special pants that wrap around pads that cover bottoms. Bodymover tools now mean that nurses need no longer lift heavy bodies but instead can strap the heavy body onto a machine that will move the body effortlessly. Of course, these tools are often necessary to prevent injury to nurses during lifting, but they are also a way of objectifying and distancing residents, and reducing the need for touching their bodies. Body control tools may be the best examples of how creative we can be as a society which cares for its elders. These tools mean that the nurse no longer needs to be present with the dementing person. Instead a computerised Panoptic eye (Foucault, 1977) is now available for installation in aged care facilities. It will warn if even one inch of the body goes near the alarm sensor pad situated on the floor beside the resident's bed or chair. The Panoptic eye also reaches into bathrooms, and informs a nurse at a distant nursing station just how much the resident's privacy is being invaded, all in the name of safety. The sound of an alarm bell alerts nurses to non-compliance or imminent escape.

The issue of resident safety is merely an excuse. There is a hidden agenda and purpose underlying the political technology of the Panoptic eye which is the imposition of tasks and certain forms of behaviour by the use of power over, and therefore control of, the residents (Foucault, 1977). A cheaper form of restraint may be found hanging behind the bodies' beds, bathroom doors or attached to the toilets: the 'belt' or 'vest' restraint. This apparatus enables nurses to tie the body into chairs or on toilets. Many nurses regard these devices very highly, because they make the resident's body 'safe'. Other bodycontrol tools include the recent proliferation of gastroenterostomy tubes: if the bodies won't eat voluntarily then we will syringe it directly into their stomachs.

One very important bodycontrol tool is the medication trolley. This trolley bulges with powerful, scientific, therapeutic, chemical inventions for behavioural control, purging, visceral cleansing and longevity. The trolley plays a dual role in that nurses may use it as a shield from the wandering dementing bodies which may want to talk to them, or worse touch them. Our tools provide us with the means of completing our principle task within the biomedical model which is to care for the patient's body. Observations of residents in these institutions are that they call out frequently, wander aimlessly in confined or locked areas, they maintain minimal or no eye contact and their facial expressions are mask-like. Many exhibit physical symptoms of the prolonged use of psychotropic medications and most are doubly incontinent. A significant number of these residents appear to be underweight. There is a high incidence of residents falling over while mobilising or when climbing out of bed (often over bedrails which have been positioned to keep them safe in bed), and of skin contusions and tears which require regular dressings. As 'busy' nurses we spend all our time managing, controlling and nursing the 'object body' of the resident. There is little emphasis or education for nurses about understanding and interpreting the unspoken language, the lived experience of the dementing resident.

The humanistic (holistic) focus of care

In units that focus on providing humanistic care within the framework of a resident-centred approach, there are no bodycare, bodymover or bodycontrol tools in sight. Staff still use lifting machines when necessary, but the rituals of body care are not the focus. Instead, the focus of care is on the needs of the whole person and their family, as perceived by the individual, at that point of time in their lives, rather than on the needs of the nursing staff and the institution. Instead of expecting the dementing person to 'function' in our world, staff enter into, and validate, the elder's experience of the world. Physical or chemical restraint are not considered as management tools and behavioural problems are 'contextually interpreted' as opposed to managed and controlled. In the disease model of dementia, the disease progression, as well as the tasks and technologies as the focus of care, are governed by objective, linear conceptions of time.

In this model 'busy' nurses spend all their time managing, controlling and nursing the 'object' body of the aged resident. Our tools provide us with the means to complete our principle task in the dementia unit, ensuring the process of disembodiment. Our ritualistic methods of using these tools guarantee we practice time thrift, time management and efficiency. The rhythm and tyranny of time control are directly related to the amount of coins in the coffers of the facilities owners and the fiscal policies of governments.

In comparison, a humanistic holistic model of the person with dementia is that of a living human being-in-the-world (Heidegger, 1962) subjectively experiencing the biological life rhythms of living, ageing and death uniquely in the present moment. Unlike the objective, third person perspective of the 'object body' or *Korper* in the biomedical or disease model, the humanistic concept of the lived body subverts the Cartesian dualism inherent in the disease model by perceiving the body as Leib or living body as the locus of experience (Leder, 1990).

A similar way of understanding this view of the body is as 'living flesh' which evokes ideas of the vulnerability and eventual decrepitude of embodiment (Parker, 1996). In these conceptualisations the mind is not decorporealised separate from the body as in Cartesian dualism – the whole self is experienced as an integrated being (Leder, 1990). The space in which dementing elders experience their life world includes both public and private. Public space includes family, nursing home and community, while private space includes their bodies as lived space, their perceptions, their feelings, their shared space, their carers, and the historical specificity of their life at the time. It is important to highlight the intersections that dementing elders encounter between supposedly separate spheres of public and private domains.

Humanistic nursing care requires a spatio-temporally relativised approach (Parker, 1988) in that lived body and lived space are entwined and integral to holistic nursing care of the resident with dementia. In units that focus on providing care within the framework of a resident centred approach, there is understanding that even in the deepest dementia process, the residents feel and still perceive. They are incarnate human beings who respond to and are motivated by feelings, needs and yearnings evoked within their corporeal and existential being. The authenticity that the world maintains for the dementing person is situated in that person's conscious awareness. But how does the nurse gain access to the inner world of the dementing person?

State of the art in dementia care

Current research suggests that many aspects of sensory perception, particularly the sense of smell, are left relatively intact during a dementing illness. One unit in the Netherlands uses various tactile props in an activity called snoezelen as a means of gaining access to the inner world of dementing elders, as well as a vehicle for staff to share their feelings with the resident (Wylie, 1994). Staff of this unit describe snoezelen as an empathic supplication to specific senses and use light, sound effects and a variety of materials for touching, smelling and tasting. In daily care, the use of dolls and hand puppets is quite common.

In a number of Swedish aged care facilities, the first sensory impressions visitors encounter are the smells of coffee and cakes baking, the colours of flowers and furnishings and the gentle rhythm of the music playing. The environment is simply that of a warm and comfortable home, whilst the atmosphere is almost ethereal. The design of these resident centred units is small and intimate, with furnishings that mirror a domestic abode rather than a hospital. They are designed with the kitchen and laundry in the centre of the lounge area as the Swedes say that domestic life revolves around family members sitting and talking whilst doing the washing and cooking.

Grooming is an essential 'task' of the carers and routines are not considered by staff: residents sleep, eat and live according to personal preferences. Here, residents maintain a high level of eye contact with their carers, respond to touch and sound, maintain healthy body weight, walk with their carers, or sit peacefully listening to music. Residents are incontinent on occasions only and in the main, staff are aware of the individual toileting patterns that each resident requires. Residents are prescribed minimal medications and chemical restraint is considered an aberrant nursing practice. The atmosphere reflects caring, comforting and embodiment of the dementing person. Staff perceive the residents as living and being rather than dementing and use their humanistic nursing skills as a creative and existential art which requires being with, rather than doing to, the dementing elder.

A number of units in Queensland use various therapies to relax residents and to increase their sensory input. Examples of these therapies include music therapy, aromatherapy and massage, and a few are using Therapeutic Touch and Healing Touch for similar reasons. Therapeutic Touch is an energy-based healing modality that is taught and practised widely as a nursing intervention (Nebauer, 1994), while Healing Touch is a group of energy-based techniques which have been developed through the American Holistic Nurses' Association (Scandrett-Hibdon, 1996). Regardless of the specific therapeutic modality or bodycare tools a resident centred unit may use, the outcome for the resident will always be determined by the craftperson who uses the tool.

Conclusion

While it is clear that government policies and fiscal restraints create tensions that impact directly and indirectly upon the type and standard of care provided for elders with dementia, nurses cannot use these imposed restraints to excuse the dehumanising care they often provide. In the final analysis, it is the values and beliefs that nurses hold about the purpose and potential of nursing and the inherent dignity and worth of each human being, and the importance of quality of life for every human being regardless of aged and medical diagnosis, that determine the way nurses choose to nurse.

Regardless of the ever present shadows of economic rationalism and continuing domination of nursing and aged care by the medical profession, there is a strong possibility that the nursing dream for a humanising, holistic focus in state of the art dementia care will remain just a dream, and aged and dementia care will continue to wallow in an outdated 'disease' model. There is a choice for nurses to make. They must choose to move from the factory to the hearth: from the cold, disembodying, controlling, 'management' of the 'object body' of the resident, to the warm, inclusive, home-like environment in which nurses creatively, bravely, sensitively and humbly enter into, and validate, the human experiences of the 'living body' of the resident with dementia.

References

Foucault M (1977) *Discipline and Punish: the Birth of the Prison*. Harmondsworth: Penguin.

Heidegger M (1962) *Being and Time*. New York: Harper and Row.

Leder D (1990) *The Absent Body*. Chicago: University of Chicago Press.

Nebauer M (1994) Healing through therapeutic touch: one person's perspective. In Gaut D and Boykin A (eds) *Caring as Healing: Renewal Through Hope*. New York: National League for Nursing.

Parker J (1996) The Body as Text and the Body as Living Flesh: Metaphors of the Body in Nursing. Unpublished paper, School of Nursing, La Trobe University, Victoria, Australia.

Parker J (1988) *Theoretical Perspectives in Nursing: from Microphysics to Hermeneutics*. Proceedings from the Third Nursing Research Forum, Lincoln Centre for Research in Nursing Practice, Melbourne, Australia.

Scandrett-Hibdon S (1996) Research Foundation. In Hover D and Kramer (eds) *Healing Touch: a Resource for Health Care Professionals*. Albany: Delmar Publishers.

Wylie K (1994) Innovative practices in dementia care. Unpublished Churchill Fellowship Report, Churchill Trust, Canberra, Australia.

Index

abuse, xv, 3, 38, 40-1, 86, 91-4, 96, 219
activities, 79, 81, 113, 140
acute care, 124, 199
acute confusional states, 130-1
ADL, 70
admission, compulsory, 16
adult placement, 89-90
advocacy, xv, 21,76, 95-101
   citizen, 97
ageism, 55, 96, 131
agencies, 69, 107-8, 110, 119, 123, 183, 194
aggression, 37, 61, 80-1, 93, 112, 140, 191, 219
agitation, 140-1, 146, 179, 221
AIDS, 193, 197, 198-203
akathesia, 141
Alzheimer's Disease, xii, 13, 28, 46-8, 51, 169,
   193, 197, 204-5
Alzheimer's Disease Society, xii, 30, 110, 121,
   194
Alzheimer's Scotland Action on Dementia, xii
anosognosia, 14
anxiety, 28, 75, 103, 135, 138, 190, 205
appointeeship, 83, 85-8
aromatherapy, 234
assessment, xv, 69, 75, 85, 103, 107, 119, 125,
   145, 152, 154-8, 184, 187, 201, 221-2, 224
attitudes, 114, 131
Australia, xiii-xv, 41, 48-54, 165, 171, 188-92,
   204-5, 234
autonomy, 57, 135, 149, 170, 218
awareness, xiv, 2-3, 5, 15

behaviour, 24, 28-9, 63, 69, 81, 93, 104, 112,
   139-40, 142, 146, 170, 176, 178, 180,188,
   199, 201-3, 212, 231-2
   challenging, 24, 63, 112, 140, 142
behavioural family therapy, 16
benefits, 83
bereavement, xvi, 64, 132, 161, 222, 224
breaks, 133; see also respite care
buildings, 114, 167, 169, 171-4
built environment, xv, 114, 182
burden (on carers), 7, 14-15, 40, 43, 212, 214
burn-out, 81

cameras, video, 146, 149
care
   acute, 124, 199
   community, 54, 62-3, 66, 84, 87, 111, 116-22,
      123-4, 126, 155, 157, 183, 208, 211, 213-14
   continuing, 52, 71
   day, 10, 14, 76, 79-80, 92, 107, 113, 121, 221
   duty of, 103, 146
   health, 10-11, 30, 54, 56, 107, 109-10, 133,
      154-5, 197, 198
   housing, xv, 58-61, 64
   legal aspects, 84, 97, 99, 142, 218
   longstay, xiv, 62-7, 76, 113, 124, 196, 208
   long-term, 52, 54-5, 115, 123, 126, 213
   management, 103, 123-8, 154; see also main
      entry management
   managers, 86, 107, 125; see also main entry
      managers
   models of, xiv, 117-21, 124-6
   packages, 14, 17, 107, 125, 221
   person-centred, 4, 195-6, 206, 218-19
   planning, 94, 102-3, 145, 155-7, 200-1
   primary, 69-71, 75, 121, 140, 186
   programme approach, 117, 119
   provision of, 43, 45, 48-50, 53, 54-6, 65, 74,
      76, 88, 97, 107, 109, 115, 117, 126
   purchasing of, 97, 109, 118, 124, 126
   residential, 19, 51, 56, 64-5, 76, 78-82, 83,
      85-6, 88, 113, 126, 165, 188, 198-203, 227,
      230-5
   respite, xv, 5, 10, 41, 76, 89-90, 93, 108, 125,
      153, 196; see also breaks
   social, 10-11, 30, 45-6, 54, 56, 76, 107,
      109-10, 133, 154-5, 197, 198
   terminal, 15, 76, 201
Care Needs Assessment Pack for Dementia
   (Carenap D), 157
caregivers, 14, 18, 39-44, 52, 209
carers, 22-3, 26, 52, 54, 58, 63, 89-90, 107,
   112-13, 124, 142, 152, 156, 196, 206, 207-9,
   211-16, 219
   burden on, 7, 14-15, 40, 43, 212, 214
   professional, 8-11; see also staff and specific
   types of caregivers
Centre for Policy on Ageing, xiii, xvii
chairs, 178-82
challenging behaviour, 24, 63, 112, 140, 142
chaplains, 225-6
charging, 83-5, 124

choice, 61, 125-6, 148, 168, 174, 180, 202, 218
citizen advocacy, 97
citizens, 94, 96-7
clinical psychology, xii
cognitive impairment, 9-10, 13, 68-9, 70, 103,
   129-32, 136, 139-43, 201
collaboration, 1, 45, 47, 71, 108, 110, 197
commissioning, 56, 109, 118, 120
communication, 2, 6, 13, 23-4, 32-6, 57-8, 94,
   100, 105, 113, 134-9, 145, 191, 202
   non-verbal, 24
communities, 116-22, 228
community care, 54, 62-3, 66, 84, 87, 111,
   116-22, 123-4, 126, 155, 157, 183, 208, 211,
   213-14
community psychiatric nurses, 71, 92-3, 108-9,
   117
complementary medicine, 200
compulsory admission, 16
confabulation, 14
confrontation, 186
confusion, 3, 9, 32, 68-9, 79, 130-1, 140, 146,
   170, 227
   acute confusional states, 130-1
consent, 17, 142-3
continuing care, 52, 71
control, 15, 38, 112, 170, 201, 219, 231-2
cookery, 5
costs, 108, 110, 123, 125
counselling, 23, 126, 196
Court of Protection, 84, 99
cultural sensivity, xiv
culture, xiii, 6, 36-7, 39, 71, 94, 105, 108, 110,
   117, 164-9, 172, 187, 196, 205
   new, xiii, 36, 206

dance therapy, 132
day care, 10, 14, 76, 79-80, 92, 107, 113, 121,
   221
death, xvi, 221-4
dementia, xvi
   frontal-type, 13
   pre-senile, 74
   prevalence of, 50
   severity of, 13-14, 78-9
   vascular, 13, 51
   see also specific diseases
Dementia Care Mapping, 1, 37, 110, 121
Dementia Services Development Centre, xiii,
   xvi
denial, 14, 160
dependants, 195
dependence, 1, 3-5, 24, 161, 177
depersonalisation, 96

depression, 13, 70, 74, 130-1
design, xv, 114, 164-9, 171-4
detection, early, 69
diagnosis, xv, 14-15, 30, 68-70, 221
   earlier/early, xv, 30, 69, 71
dignity, 15-16, 49, 106, 146, 149, 234
disability, xv, 96
disabling (care-related), xiv, 96, 143, 181
discharge from hospital, 107-8, 124
discrimination, 96, 131
disease, 51-2, 125, 131, 138, 146, 218, 230-2
   prevention of, 54
   see also specific diseases
district nurses, 52
domiciliary services, 85, 109, 113, 125
Downs Syndrome, 194
drama therapy, 132
driving, 16
drugs, 15, 55, 129-31
   neuroleptic, xv, 130, 139-44
   see also medication; polypharmacy
duty of care, 103, 146
dystonias, 141

earlier diagnosis, xv, 69
early diagnosis, 30, 71
early detection, 69
early onset, 21, 74, 193
education, 17, 22, 30, 51, 53, 70
   psychoeducation, 132
electroconvulsive therapy (ECT), 131
empathy, 38-9, 135, 174
empowerment, 34, 95, 147-8, 155-6, 180, 186;
   see also power
enduring power of attorney, 16, 84-5
environment, xv-xvi, 48, 57-8, 64-6, 79-81, 103,
   105, 112-14, 137, 146-8, 162, 164-8, 170,
   175-6, 182, 197, 199-201, 203, 233
   built, xv, 114, 182
ethics, 99, 142-3, 148-9, 156
ethnicity, xiii, 100
   minority ethnic groups, xiii, 100, 120, 165-8,
   196, 228
Europe, 68-70, 78-82, 234
European Alzheimer Clearing House, 46-8
European Union Public Health Policy, 47
evaluation, xvi, 1, 135, 157, 174, 194, 207-11,
   214

families, xvi, 7-12, 15, 19, 39-44, 71, 75, 105,
   123, 125, 222
   therapy, 132
fiction, xii
finances, xv, 83-9

fire, 104-5
food, 60, 79, 172, 175-7
friends and friendship, 60
frontal-type dementia, 13
furniture, 80, 114, 168, 178-82

gender, 60-1, 123, 172, 212
General Health Questionnaires, 211
general practice and practitioners, xv, 53, 67-72,
  75, 93, 108, 117-18, 121, 124-5, 183, 186,
  221
genetics, 75
government, central, 124, 225, 234
grief, 32, 64, 160-1, 222
grounded theory, 26
group homes, 78-82
group work, xiv
groups, xiv, 57-62, 98, 132, 135, 137
  homogeneity of, 60
  minority ethnic, xiii, 100, 120, 165-8, 196,
  228
  support, 8, 21, 30, 92-3, 132, 208
  treatment, 208
guardianship, 16, 99
guilt, 39-44, 92

hallucinations, 69, 130, 143, 202
health, 69
  care, 10-11, 30, 54, 56, 107, 109-10, 133,
  154-5, 197, 198
  services, 54, 91
  trusts, 54, 56, 109, 111, 117-22
Health Advisory Service, 120
helplessness, learned, 57-8
HIV see AIDS
holistic approach, xvi, 157, 198-203, 230-5
home, xv, 76, 79, 85, 87, 103-5, 148, 164-5,
  170-1
  helps, 78-9, 91-2
homogeneity (of groups), 60
hospices, 15, 199
hospitals, 62-7, 75, 107, 124, 143, 175-6
  discharge from, 107-8, 124
hostels, 50, 165-8, 171, 188-91
housing, 147, 171-4, 196, 198-203
  care housing, xv, 58-61, 64

identity, 34, 134, 161-2
income, 109
incontinence, 9, 146, 181-2, 202, 231, 233
independence, 16, 57, 64, 88, 149, 176, 214
individuality, 57, 106, 149, 225
infra-red systems, 146, 149
inequality, 56

in-patients, 120-1
insight, xiv, 2-3, 13-18, 32, 132
inspection (of services), 45-6
institutionalisation, 3, 16, 42, 126, 213-14
institutions, 41, 63, 65-6, 78-9, 94, 126,
  211-12
insurance, private, 55-6
interdependence, 1, 4-5
interventions, xiv-xv, 10-11, 30, 60, 65, 69, 104,
  123, 131, 142, 146, 190-1, 199, 207-8, 211,
  214, 221
Invalid Care Allowance, 21

Jacob-Creutzfeldt Syndrome, 51
joint work, xv, 106-11, 125
Journal of Dementia Care xiii, 205-6

keyworkers, 120
kinship, 212

language, 24, 134, 196
learned helplessness, 57-8
learning difficulties, 63, 139, 197
legal aspects of care, 84, 97, 99, 142, 218
legislation, 7, 16, 96, 99, 108, 117
less developed countries, xiii
Lewy Body dementia, 76
life histories, 37, 75, 135
life stories, xv, 102, 149-53, 159-63
local authorities, 45-6, 79, 83-9, 126, 213
longitudinal studies, 40
longstay care, xiv, 62-7, 76, 113, 124, 196, 208
long-term care, 52, 54-5, 115, 123, 126, 213

management, 65, 71, 74, 76, 85, 114, 116-20,
  122, 123-7; see also care management
managers, 6, 85-7, 91, 102-3, 107, 115, 116, 118,
  121-2, 126, 137, 183, 185 see also care
  managers
marriage, 15, 37-8, 212-13
meals, 79, 104
mealtimes, xvi, 175-8
medication, 69, 108, 126, 142, 201-2, 231, 233;
  see also drugs; polypharmacy
medicine, complementary, 200
memories, 3, 137, 160, 205, 228
memory, 23, 30, 68-9, 89, 103, 160-2, 204, 219,
  221-2, 225, 227, 229
Mental Health Act Commission, 120
mental health services, 91
mental health teams, 116-22, 124, 196
metaphor, 3, 23, 159-60, 162
minority ethnic groups, xiii, 100, 120, 165-8,
  196, 228

models of care, xiv, 117-21, 124-6
multidisciplinary approach, 17, 45, 107, 116-22,
    154, 183-7, 196-7, 199
music therapy, 132, 234
narrative, 3, 32, 159-63
National Audit Office, 84
National Health Service, 45, 54, 56
National Health Service and Community Care
    Act (1990), 83, 96, 107-9
negotiations, 122, 202
neighbours, 71, 156, 167
neuroleptic drugs, xv, 130, 139-44
neurology, xiv, 39, 70-1, 75
new culture, xiii, 36, 206
non-fiction, xii
non-verbal communication, 24
normalisation, 8-9, 11, 28-9
nurses, xii, 68, 71, 92-4, 97, 108-9, 117, 125-6,
    183, 188, 200, 230-2, 234
    community psychiatric nurses, 71, 92-3,
        108-9, 117
    district, 52
nursing homes, 50, 56, 64, 76, 79-80, 83, 85, 88,
    94, 113, 124, 126, 139-40, 143, 171, 188-9,
    199, 222
nutrition, 104-5

observation, 156
occupational therapy, 117, 183-4, 188
onset, early, 21, 74, 193
orders, short procedure, 84-5
outcomes, 27, 53, 105, 190-2, 208-9, 234

packages of care, 14, 17, 107, 125, 221
paranoia, 13, 69, 74-5
Parkinson's Disease and Parkinsonian effects,
    141
passive infra-red systems, 146, 149
performance indicators, 53
person-centred care and planning, 4, 195-6,
    206, 218-19
personality, 13
personhood, 10, 23, 36-9, 64, 96, 135, 137, 146,
    149
pharmacology see drugs; medication;
    polypharmacy
philosophy, 23, 146, 148-9, 188, 200-1, 203,
    214, 218
Pick's Disease, 51, 194
placement, adult, 89-90
poetry, xii, 32-5, 162
policies, xiv, 7, 54-6, 86, 88, 234
polypharmacy, 140
power, 5, 94, 220; see also empowerment

power of attorney see enduring power of
    attorney
preferences, 115, 176
pre-senile dementia, 74
prevalence (of dementia), 50
prevention (of disease), 54
primary care, 69-71, 75, 121, 140, 186
privacy, 19, 140, 146, 149, 166, 172, 231
private insurance, 55-6
private sector, 45, 55, 88, 107
problem-solving, 27
professional carers, 8-11; see also staff and
    specific types of caregivers
prognosis, 8, 14
provision of care, 43, 45, 48-50, 53, 54-6, 65, 74,
    76, 88, 97, 107, 109, 115, 117, 126
psychiatrists, xii, 71, 74, 129
psychiatry, xv, 75-7, 118-19, 129-34
psychoeducation, 132
psychogeriatric services, 51
psychologists and psychology, xii, 117
    clinical, xii
psychoses, 16, 74
psychotherapy, xv, 23, 57, 75, 159-63, 196
purchasing (of care), 97, 109, 118, 124, 126

quality assurance, 52-3

rationality, xiv
reality orientation, xii, 16, 132, 201
receivership, 84-5, 87-8
reciprocity, 8, 42-3, 135, 218
recruitment, 111-15
regulation, 56
rehabilitation, xiv, 51, 54
relationships, xiv, xvi, 8, 10-11, 41-3, 58, 75-6,
    90, 92, 95, 113, 125, 134-5, 152, 164, 203,
    207-8, 212-14, 218-220
reminiscence, xv, 132, 135-8
research and researchers, xvi, 17, 24, 26, 64-5,
    76, 131, 178, 194, 204, 207-11, 213-14, 225,
    228
residential care, 19, 51, 56, 64-5, 76, 78-82, 83,
    85-6, 88, 113, 126, 165, 188, 198-203, 227,
    230-5
residential staff, xii, 79-81, 230-5
residents, 58-61, 79-82, 165-6, 200-1, 231,
    233-4
respite care, xv, 5, 10, 41, 76, 89-90, 93, 108,
    125, 153, 196; see also breaks
Revised Elderly Persons Disability Scale
    (REPDS), 145
rights, 91, 94-6, 99, 146, 219
risk, 94, 96, 102-6, 141, 200, 202

Royal College of Nursing, 56
rummaging, 104

safety, 147-8, 176, 231
screening, 68, 70, 125
seating *see chairs*
self-determination, 9, 91, 218
services, xiv-xv, 7, 14, 21, 23, 30, 45-6, 49, 51-2,
    73, 76, 87-8, 92-3, 107-8, 111, 116-22, 154-5,
    207-11, 213
  domiciliary, 85, 109, 113, 125
  health, 54, 91
  inspection of, 45-6
  mental health, 91
  psychogeriatric, 51
  sitter, 14
  social, 45-6, 71, 87-8, 91, 107, 109, 111,
    117-18, 120, 122
  support, 21, 49, 92-3
severity (of dementia), 13-14, 78-9
sex and sexuality, xvi, 217-21
short procedure orders, 84-5
side effects, 129-30, 139-41
sitter services, 14
size (of teams), 118; *see small*
sleep, 104, 108
sleeplessness, 75
small, 171-174; *see design*
smell (sense of), 175, 233
snoezelen approach, 121, 233
social care, 10-11, 30, 45-6, 54, 56, 76, 107,
    109-10, 133, 154-5, 197, 198
social construction, 25, 29
social interaction, 57-62, 177, 180
social security, 54
social services, 45-6, 71, 87-8, 91, 107, 109, 111,
    117-18, 120, 122
social workers, xii, 21, 71, 90, 93, 97, 117, 119,
    125-6, 183-4, 186
solicitors, 83-4
specialists, 115
speech, 14, 227
spirituality, xvi, 174, 202, 225-9
spouses, 14-15, 18, 212-13
staff, xii, 3, 6, 41, 45, 58, 60, 62-7, 70, 79-81,
    85-6, 88, 94, 103, 108, 110-22, 125, 206, 219
  residential, xii, 79-81, 230-5
staffing levels, 177
status, 184, 218
stigma, 3, 10, 21, 65
strain, 40, 42
stress, 7, 15, 17, 81, 211-13
structure, 145, 191
suicide, 15

support groups, 8, 21, 30, 92-3, 132, 208
support services, 21, 49, 92-3
symbolism, 24, 190, 227

teams, 74, 80, 115, 116-22, 124-7, 183, 185-6,
    199-200, 203
  mental health, 116-22, 124, 196
  size of, 118
technology, xv, 144-9, 231
tagging, 146
tardive dyskinesia, 141
telephones, 125, 145, 148
terminal care, 15, 76, 201
therapies, 16, 23, 57, 65, 75-6, 121, 129-34,
    159-63, 234
  aromatherapy, 234
  dance, 132
  drama, 132
  electroconvulsive (ECT), 131
  family therapy, 16, 132
  music, 132, 234
  occupational, 117, 183-4, 188
  psychotherapy, xv, 23, 57, 75, 159-63, 196
  validation, xii
toilets, 114, 164
training, xvi, 17, 24, 30, 51, 53, 70, 86, 88, 110,
    126, 177, 183-7, 188-92
transport, 96
treatment groups, 208

uniqueness, xvi, 36-9, 137
users (of care), 125

validation therapy, xii
vascular dementia, 13, 51
video cameras, 146, 149
'voice', 4, 22-5, 100
volunteers, 54, 97

wandering, 9, 105, 146, 178, 231
weight (body), 181, 231
welfare, 54, 56, 107
wellbeing, 56, 57, 61, 88, 112, 180, 194, 206,
    212-13, 220

young people, xiv, xvi, 18-22
younger people, 74, 193-203